SEX SENSE
CANADIAN CONTRACEPTION GUIDE

PREFACE
AND ACKNOWLEDGEMENTS

We believe that contraception is a very important key to not only sexual health, but to health and happiness in general. This book is a practical guide on how to be safely sexual or, how one student who worked on the development of the book put it: "How to have a blast while staying out of trouble!"

You may ask yourself why the Society of Obstetricians and Gynaecologists of Canada decided to publish a book on contraception because you have probably already seen a variety of pamphlets and brochures on this subject. We felt that we should share with you the experience and knowledge we have as a medical organization. Canadians who want to learn more about their health and about the choices they have to stay healthy should have access to a professional and complete source of information.

The text is based on the Canadian Consensus Conference on Contraception. What is that? Medical professionals with a special interest in sexual health from across Canada got together and came up with guidelines to help other health care professionals serve you better. These guidelines were published in 1998. They are based on evidence, on the results of clinical studies.

This book is about everything you will ever want to know about contraception. Each method is presented in a question and answer format including important questions like, "How effective is a chosen method in preventing pregnancy and sexually transmitted infections and HIV?"

This guide should support you in choosing a contraceptive method that best suits your health and lifestyle.

We owe thanks to the members and chairs of the Contraception Consensus Committee, who provided the groundwork for the manuscript.

Special thanks to the many people who helped to make this book possible:

The design team from the Department of Design Art at Concordia University in Montreal (seven dedicated and skilled students and and their professor), who created the artistic part of what you have in your hands now. Thanks also to the Visual Arts Mac Labs for providing computer and printing facilities.

The people who took the time and patience to revise the entire manuscript. Thank you for all the comments, advice and great suggestions: Richard Boroditsky (MD), Edith Guilbert (MD), Terry O'Grady (MD), André B. Lalonde (MD), Lydia Sharman (PHD), Christiane Ménard, Bonnie Johnson, Glenna Elhilali, Yehia Nachabé, Natacha Vairo, Tamzyn Berman, Tevis Houston, Kajin Goh.

Thanks also to the many people and organizations who provided input on individual chapters.

Planned Parenthood Federation of Canada who provided us with information and addresses of people to turn to for questions and support regarding contraception. You'll find these addresses in the address section at the end of the book.

Janssen-Ortho Inc. who provided the results of the 1998 Canadian Contraception Study. In this study, 1,599 Canadians in the age group 15-44 were asked about their use of contraceptives. It will be published in the Canadian Journal of Human Sexuality in the year 2000.

Durex Canada who supplied us with the results of the "1999 Global Sex Survey - A Youth Perspective." In this study the attitudes and sexual behaviours of 16-21 year-olds in 14 countries were examined. The survey included 4,200 sexually active and non-active young females and males. For more information visit their website: www.durex.com

INTRODUCTION
SEX AND HEALTH - ALL ABOUT A WINNING TEAM

Sex is fun, sex is necessary. And let's face it, for some people it is more important than for others. What is true for everybody: it touches your body and emotions and can affect your health like no other activity. It can make you ecstatic, happy, want to dance on the moon and reach for the stars. And it can make you sad; it can make you sick. It can also lead to pregnancy! Don't get us wrong here. Expecting a baby might be the greatest thing for many couples, but it can also mean disaster to others.

Where did all the fun go?
Why is it all so complicated? Why can't we just have fun? Simply because it takes two to tango and because times have changed drastically. In the good old days you felt attracted to somebody and you had sex. No big deal. Nowadays youth grow up with the warning of HIV, sexually transmitted infections (STIs), and sexual violence. Where did all the fun go?

Let us tell you, it can still be there. But fun might need a bit more planning than it used to. This book helps you to stay out of trouble while enjoying the pleasurable side of sex. This handy guide discusses all contraceptive methods available in Canada. We will look at how they work, how effective they are, how well they protect you from STIs and how much they cost. At the beginning of each chapter, "In a nutshell" gives a summary of the method. If it doesn't spark your interest, forget about that chapter and go to the next method.

There are many myths about contraception. This book wants to lift the fog and provide you with fact-based information. The text has short paragraphs, some of which are headed by a question. You can select the sections you are interested in and skip the ones that go into too much detail. This guide will help you to make an informed choice about contraception. YOU are important. Take care of yourself. Have fun but protect yourself. Stay healthy and be happy and you'll have it all!

To do "it" is not everything
Most of the stuff we are talking about in this book involves "it," to have intercourse. This should not give the impression that it is the focal point of having sex. There are a million ways to find pleasure, fulfilment and excitement while having sex, be it with intercourse or without. However, since contraception and protection against STIs and HIV are directly related to the exchange of body fluids, we are focusing on this part of sex. That is why we do not talk a whole lot about other ways of showing affection, passion and desire.

Contraception is also about relationships. A relationship can combine love and sex, it can also be loving without being sexual, and it can also be sexual without love being involved. How is your relationship with your partner? Are you talking about sex? How comfortable are you in sharing a responsibility, like the protection against pregnancy? You should spend time thinking about these questions before making choices.

You have rights. Use them!

Sexuality is a normal expression of life. The choice of a contraceptive method is more than an intellectual choice. It involves feelings towards sexuality, sense of self, your feelings towards your partner and many other emotions. Be responsible and show respect to your partner.

We also provide you with addresses, websites and phone numbers of where to turn to with questions regarding contraception, STIs and unintended pregnancy. Get started, have fun reading and don't forget to write down any questions that you might have. You should discuss them with your health care provider.

This book cannot replace the care and support that you can get from medical professionals when you have a personal appointment. Family planning clinics, family physicians, gynaecologists, pharmacists and nurses at schools and universities are there for you. The only thing you have to do is to approach them and they will help you.

KEEP A FEW THINGS IN MIND WHEN CHOOSING A CONTRACEPTIVE:

It is your right to protect yourself from pregnancy and diseases.

It is your right to enjoy yourself.

It is your right to determine when, with whom, how and where you want to have sex.

It is your right to delay sexual activity.

It is your right to make your own choices.

**1998 Canadian Contraception Study:
USE OF CONTRACEPTIVES**

- Among single young women who had sexual intercourse during the past six months, only 60% of 15-17 year-olds and 68% of 18-24 year-olds always used a method of contraception.

- Familiarity with the range of available contraceptives has dropped steadily and consistently during the past twenty years.

TABLE OF CONTENTS

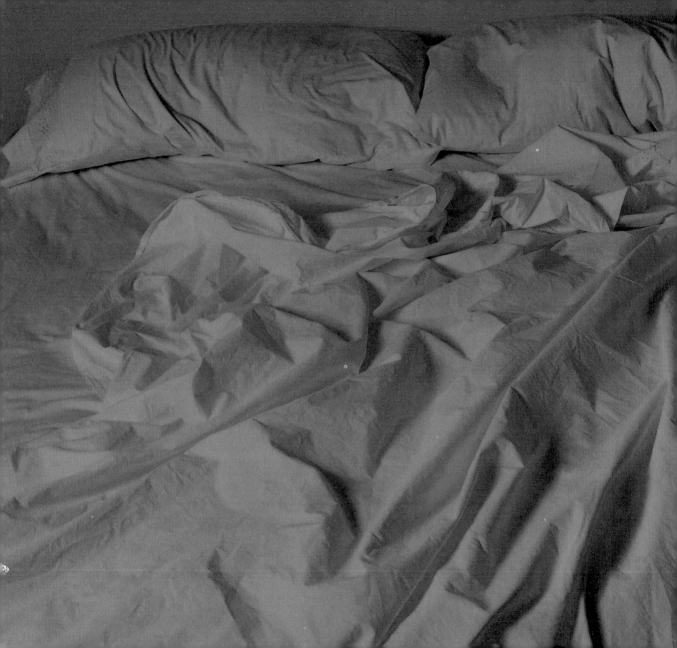

THE BASICS

A REFRESHER ON REPRODUCTION

You think you know all about it? Even if you do, here is a refresher course. We will give you some facts on how this business of reproduction works.

Puberty changes the male and female bodies making them physically able to reproduce in order to keep the human race alive. In this book we won't talk about the emotional issues that go along with puberty, however, this is a very exciting time, changing lives forever.

THE BODY AND THE HORMONES

Most of us are equipped to have kids. Of course there are exceptions, for example when individuals suffer from certain conditions which cause infertility. In addition to organs such as the liver, heart and lungs, we have reproductive organs and we produce hormones inside our bodies. They are courier substances within the blood, which convey messages from one organ to another. There are many different types of hormones. One group, sex hormones, controls reproduction.

The most important sex hormones in the female body are estrogen and progesterone. The male hormones are called androgens. The most important androgen is testosterone. Androgens are not only found in males and estrogens in females. Men carry female hormones and women carry male hormones as well.

Let's look at the difference between the male and female reproductive organs. When choosing a method of contraception these "little" differences actually make a big difference.

The male
From the reproductive point of view the major differences between males and females are:

- Starting at puberty men can make babies basically anytime (provided they ejaculate).
- Sperm can stay alive in a woman's uterus up to three days.
- Men are able to father children almost until the end of their lives.
- They do not have a cycle to regulate fertility like women do.
- Men need to reach orgasm and have to ejaculate to reproduce.

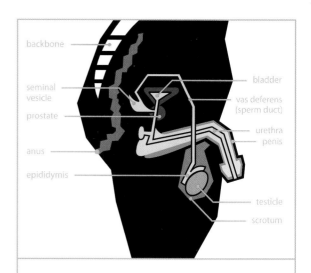

There are interior (epididymis, vas deferens, prostate, urethra) and exterior reproductive organs (penis, scrotum holding the testicles or testes).

Sperm production - how men produce babies
Sperm production starts with the onset of puberty at an average age of 13 years and lasts throughout the life of a man. The sure sign for a young man that he is able to reproduce is that his erection is followed by an ejaculation. This is of course only "physically speaking." Emotionally, you might be very far from being ready to take the responsibility of becoming a father. Sperm, more precisely spermatozoa, are produced by the testicles, which are glands within the scrotum.

The scrotum functions like a thermostat regulating the temperature of the testicles. If you're a male then you know that the scrotum becomes smaller and more wrinkled when you enter a cold pool. The scrotum contracts to bring the testicles closer to the body to keep them warm. The testicles produce hormones and sperm. Sperm production is an ongoing process. It takes about 70 days for one sperm to mature.

Let's have a look at how sperm actually grow. At the beginning of the process sperm form in the testicles, then travel through the epididymis. After that the sperm reach the vas deferens, they are stored there until ejaculation occurs. The prostate gland produces a liquid that helps sperm to survive after leaving the male body. During ejaculation, spermatozoa and liquid from the prostate and other glands make a mix while traveling through the urethra. This mix is called semen. The urethra is a tube that also connects to the bladder for passing urine. During sexual excitement this connection is interrupted so that semen does not come into contact with urine.

A sperm has the ability to swim and travel on its own. It has an oval-shaped head and a tail that serves as a propeller. Sperm carry the genetic properties of the male and can unite with the female egg to produce an embryo, which after two months of pregnancy becomes a fetus, and later becomes a baby.

Survival of the fittest
Spermatozoa are very fragile and their chances of survival are very low. This is the reason why the testicles of each individual produce millions of them each day. The milky or creamy looking ejaculate consists of hundreds of millions of sperm, but only a few of them will survive the journey through the female vagina to the fallopian tube where the female egg is waiting to meet a sperm. Out of those few only one will actually enter the egg and fertilize it.

Sperm, although it is very fragile, can also be very persistent. Occasionally pregnancy can occur without intercourse. This is called "splash pregnancy." Sperm have been known to move very quickly from outside the vagina into the uterus. After intercourse sperm can survive a couple of days in the uterus.

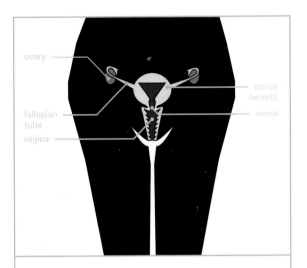

ovary

uterus (womb)

fallopian tube

cervix

vagina

The female body has interior and exterior reproductive organs. The interior organs are: cervix, uterus, fallopian tubes (8-10 cm) and ovaries. The cervix is the entrance to the uterus. The exterior ones are: mons pubis, clitoris, opening of the vagina (6-10 cm), inner and outer lips, and hymen (not shown in this illustration).

The female
Remember what we said earlier about the differences between the sexes? Here are the little differences that make up a female:

- A woman is able to have children from the time she begins to menstruate (around 12 years) to the onset of menopause (around 52 years).
- A woman can only conceive if intercourse occurs during the four days surrounding ovulation.
- A woman has a menstrual cycle that determines her fertility.
- A female egg can only be fertilized by male semen in a limited time frame.

- A woman can become pregnant without being sexually aroused and reaching orgasm.
- A woman could be a virgin and still get pregnant (splash pregnancy).

Puberty: when hormones start working overtime

Already at birth the female body is equipped with a bank account of 300-400,000 egg cells which are located in the ovaries. Of this large amount only 300-500 will be released during the reproductive years of a woman's life. Starting between the ages of 8-10, hormone production rises and makes the body change from a child to a young adult. The first menstruation, between 11-14, is a sure sign that the body is preparing to have children. This is of course only "physically speaking." Emotionally, you might be very far from being ready to have children of your own.

From puberty on:

- The female produces one egg every month in the left or the right ovary.
- This egg is released (ovulation) to start its journey to the uterus through one of the fallopian tubes.
- The body prepares for a possible pregnancy.

Keep in mind that we're talking about the usual stuff here. Of course there are exceptions such as the production of more than one egg which might lead to two or more babies. This all happens due to the amazing teamwork between the hormones and organs. These things go on over and over again each month and this is what we call the female cycle.

The amazing female cycle

The cycle covers a time frame of 23-35 days. The average cycle lasts 28 days. The first day of the cycle is the first day of menstruation. The last day of the cycle is the last day before the following menstruation. Cycle lengths vary individually and they are not always regular. Stress, for example, can also disturb the cycle. After the first menstruation, it normally takes 1-3 years until a woman gets a regular cycle.

During the first 14 days of the cycle (usually, but depending on cycle length) an egg is ripening. A hormone in the brain, which is called follicle stimulating hormone (FSH), stimulates the ripening process. The coat around the egg produces estrogen. This most important female hormone makes the lining of the uterus grow to form a nutritious and secure bedding for the egg to settle into after fertilization.

Approximately at day 14 of a 28-day cycle, an egg is ripe. Another hormone in the brain, which is called luteinizing hormone (LH), gives the impulse for the egg to emerge from the ovary and be taken up by the fallopian tube. This important event is called ovulation. This is also the most fertile time of the month for a woman to get pregnant. The egg then travels through the fallopian tube to the uterus. The journey takes about seven days. In the meantime another important hormone produced in the ovary, progesterone, is preparing the uterus for a pregnancy by securing a sufficient blood supply and by preventing the uterus from contracting and losing a fertilized egg.

Fertilization most often occurs in the 6-12 hours after ovulation. Fertilization happens when sperm enters the egg and starts the growth of the embryo. Two cells divide and become four, the four cells divide and become eight, etc. By the time the cluster of cells reaches the uterus and settles down into the lining of the uterus, it has become an embryo.

This settling down is called implantation. It takes about seven days from fertilization to implantation. The rise of estrogen and progesterone in the blood stream of the woman, along with the pregnancy hormone human chorionic gonadotropin (HCG) from cells surrounding the embryo, signals pregnancy. From now on the female body occupies itself with the growth of the embryo and stops the cycle until a few weeks after the baby is born. This is the reason why women cannot conceive again while they are pregnant. A woman can only have one pregnancy at a time but this does not exclude the possibility of having more than one embryo or fetus at a time, e.g. twins.

The rise in estrogen and progesterone signals to the ovaries: Do not produce any more eggs for now. We have to take care of this embryo first! A pregnancy test would be positive about 14 days after ovulation. If no fertilization of the egg occurs, the production of progesterone stops. So does the production of estrogens. The message is basically: We do not have a fertilized egg to produce an embryo this month, so stop all the preparations and start all over again! The end of the story is that the lining of the uterus, which was supposed to be the bed for the fertilized egg, is no longer necessary. The same applies to the egg, which did not get fertilized. The body rids itself of this bedding and the egg by bleeding. This is known as the period or menstruation.

The link to contraception

This was a brief description of what's happening with our bodies when it comes to reproduction. What does this have to do with contraception then? Remember we were talking about the principles of contraception:

- Hormonal methods make the body believe the ovaries produce hormones while they are, in fact, resting.
- Barrier methods prevent sperm and egg from meeting each other.
- Chemical methods (spermicides) destroy sperm upon contact.
- Surgical methods interrupt the transportation route of eggs or sperm.
- Emergency contraception: a hormonal reaction creates unfavourable conditions for egg and sperm to meet.

1998 Canadian Contraception Study: LOOK AFTER YOURSELF

- Of all Canadian women aged 15-45, 28% reported that they had had an unintended pregnancy.

- Of women who have had intercourse during the past six months and used a method of contraception, 44% used the condom, 43% used the pill, 25% used female or male sterilization, 9% used withdrawal, 3% used the IUD, 2% used "rhythm", 2% used Depo-Provera, and 1% used the emergency OC method.

DID YOU KNOW?

- 25% of young women who have intercourse without using a method of birth control will become pregnant within one month.
- 85% will become pregnant within one year.

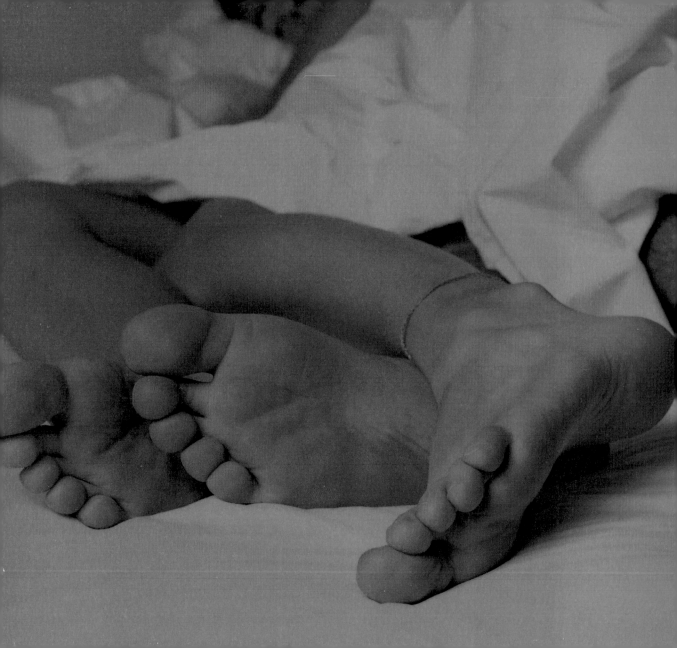

SAFER SEX

WHY CAN'T IT JUST BE FUN?

In this chapter we will talk about safer sex. Ever since HIV and AIDS entered our lives in the early 1980s we have heard a lot about this subject. More and more young people are diagnosed with an STI (Sexually Transmitted Infection), including HIV, in Canada every day. Sometimes you might ask yourself why can't sex just be fun? We don't want to scare you or convince you to abstain from sex altogether. We want to make you aware of some facts. After studying them you can make up your mind for yourself whether you want to practice safer sex or not.

WHAT SAFER SEX MEANS IN OUR BOOK:

▶ While having sex, go "Dutch Treat" and use double protection!

▶ Protect yourself from sexually transmitted infections including HIV/AIDS.

▶ Protect yourself from unintended pregnancy.

HOW DO YOU ACHIEVE ALL OF THAT?
By avoiding the exchange of blood or body fluids.

IT'S ALL UP TO YOU
In every chapter of this book we talk about the safety of each method in protecting you and your partner from STIs and HIV/AIDS. You do not have to be a rocket scientist to find out that there are basically only two methods at this time that protect against STIs and HIV.

- The male latex condom (and soon the polyurethane male condom when it comes on the Canadian market).
- The female condom.

For maximum protection both kinds of condoms should be used with a spermicide.

Why "safer" sex rather than "safe" sex?
We call our recommendations "safer" sex, rather than safe sex. Why is this so? The only safe sex is no sex, just fantasies, or abstinence. For more on that flip to Chapter 6. Sex with a condom is not absolutely safe, it is only safer. The latex condom has its disadvantages. It does not cover the whole genital area of both partners. During skin to skin contact the transmission of viruses, which are responsible for herpes and genital warts (HPV), can still be transmitted from one person to the other.

Condoms are still the best bet!
If you want to practice safer sex, avoid the exchange of fluids by engaging in other pleasuring activities. Condoms and spermicides are still your best bet. Even if you choose a method other than the male or female condom, you'll still have to use it in combination with either the male latex or the female condom to protect yourself and your partner from infections.

In this chapter we cover the following subjects:

- Some facts about STIs and HIV.
- Safer sex recommendations.
- Are you at risk of catching an STI or HIV?
  A questionnaire helps you to find out for yourself.

THE GOOD NEWS:
MOST STIs CAN BE CURED.
OTHERS CAN BE CONTROLLED.

THE BAD NEWS:
SOME, LIKE HIV, CAN KILL YOU.

Blood could come from wounds in your mouth, on your lips, or anywhere on your body, menstrual blood, from sharing injection needles, or from needles for piercing or tattoos.

Body fluids are semen, sperm, pre-ejaculatory fluid (fluid which comes out of the penis during sexual arousal), saliva (especially when there is a cut in or around your mouth), breast milk and vaginal fluids.

Some facts about STIs and HIV

Sexually transmitted infections are troublesome. They can be passed from person to person through sexual activity and exchange of body fluids. It is absolutely wrong to believe that it is a disgrace to get infected, that it means you have a "loose" character or are not a clean person. It can happen to any sexually active person (movie actors, pop stars and other heroes included!). It is a fact that STIs are most common in young adults under the age of 25. Women in the age group 15-19 have the highest rate of STIs in Canada. This is especially true for chlamydia and gonorrhea. But, basically anyone who is sexually active can get infected.

Infertility can be a consequence of untreated STIs. It seems unfair but women suffer more severe long-term consequences including infertility, pelvic inflammatory disease, ectopic pregnancy, chronic pelvic pain, and cervical cancer. Women are also less likely to see a doctor if they are infected because many STIs in women have no symptoms and the infection is more difficult to diagnose. STIs spread with:

- The exchange of body fluids is the most common way to pass on an infection, no matter whether they are bacterial or viral infections.
- Skin to skin contact is another way to pass on certain infections. Herpes and HPV are spread by skin to skin contact and a condom may not fully protect you.
- Infected women who are pregnant can unknowingly pass some infections to their babies during pregnancy and at birth.
- Infected mothers can unknowingly pass the HIV virus through their breast milk.

No symptoms. No worry? Not quite!

STIs and HIV can affect anybody. STIs are unpredictable because you or your partner might not have any symptoms. Symptoms can show weeks, months or even years later. In the case of HIV it is possible that 15 years pass before the infection actually leads to AIDS. You can spread the infection without even knowing it because even though you may be infected, you may not have had any symptoms. You cannot tell by looking at or touching someone whether that person is infected. When somebody is clean and good-looking it does not mean he/she is not infected. You only know when you get a test done or when the disease is at a later stage. If you are sexually active, having intercourse or starting a sexual relationship with someone new, you and your partner should go for STI testing. When? A test before having sex and another test 3-6 months later.

1999 Global Sex Survey: DO YOU HAVE FEARS RELATED TO SEX?

- Fear of HIV and other STIs has the most impact with 16-21 year-olds, regardless of gender.

- 45% of respondents said HIV and STIs are their biggest fears.

- In second place comes unintended pregnancy: 32% of female respondents, 18% of male respondents stated that as their biggest fear.

HERE IS A SHORT OVERVIEW OF THE MOST COMMON STIs:

Bacterial infections
These STIs are treated with antibiotics prescribed by your physician or at a clinic.

Chlamydia The most common STI in Canada. Usually no or few symptoms. Can lead to pelvic inflammatory disease, ectopic pregnancy (a pregnancy outside the uterus) and sterility in women and men.

Trichomoniasis A type of vaginitis, which is an inflammation of the vagina. Only women can get this disease but men can spread this infection.

Gonorrhoea Can lead to sterility in women and men, to arthritis, and in rare cases can affect your heart, brain and spinal cord.

Syphilis This disease can affect the whole body (also the health of an unborn child). It can, over many years, lead to paralysis, heart disease, brain damage, and even death.

Viral infections
These STIs are more difficult to treat because viruses cause them. After infection the virus might stay in your body forever.

HIV / AIDS HIV is the virus that causes AIDS. This disease destroys the immune system. Modern drugs help to prolong the life of people living with the virus but there is no cure available. Symptoms may show as late as 15 years after becoming infected. Symptoms include: swollen glands in the neck, groin or armpit, unexplained diarrhoea, nightsweats and weight loss.

Genital warts / HPV The warts on the skin in the genital area can be so small that they are hard to detect. Warts can also be on the walls of the vagina and cervix. Human papillomaviruses (HPV) can lead to various diseases, including cervical cancer. A variety of treatments are available, such as surgical removal of the warts. It is important to have regular Pap smears because an infection can be invisible.

Hepatitis B It starts as an inflammation of the liver and can develop into a serious liver disease. Hepatitis usually shows symptoms such as yellowing of the skin and eyes and flu-like symptoms. The good news: Hepatitis B is the only STI for which a vaccine is available.

Herpes A virus that causes blisters on the skin, especially on the penis, on the entrance of the vagina, and on the lips. It also causes cold sores in the mouth and on the gums. Can cause infections in an unborn baby. No cure available but treatment with prescription drugs.

If there are symptoms, hurry to see your doctor or go to a clinic!

If there are symptoms, they could be the following:

- Unusual discharge (amount, odour, colour) from penis, vagina or rectum.
- Pain in genitals or lower body.
- Itching, sores, bumps, rash on genitals or anus.
- Unusual bleeding, bleeding after intercourse.
- A bad smell.
- Swollen glands.

Safer sex recommendations

Here are a few ways to practice safer sex. The safest sex is abstinence; the second safest sex is sex between partners in a mutually monogamous relationship who are not infected (proven by tests!)."Mutually monogamous" is a complicated term for a simple thing. It means: you have sex with no one else but your partner and your partner has sex with no one else but you. This is the ideal situation that may not always be possible. Here are the steps:

- Talk to your partner about safer sex, testing, and define your own boundaries in your sexual relationship.
- Use a condom and spermicide for all types of sexual activity, especially for intercourse.
- Use a spermicide with all barrier methods.
- Engage in sexual activities that do not necessarily lead to intercourse.
- If there is any doubt about you or your partner being infected, then it is best to practice safer sex until you are absolutely sure.
- Do not share needles for drugs, tattoos, piercing, steroids.

Basic guidelines for safer sex

The most important thing to keep in mind: No exchange of blood and body fluids!

Kissing French kissing should be avoided immediately after brushing your teeth, after using dental floss, or if either partner has sores in the mouth. Dry kissing is safer. Kissing the partner's genitals can spread STIs.

Masturbation Masturbation alone or with one or more partners is safe. Avoid any exchange of blood or body fluids, especially if there are any openings in the skin.

Oral Sex It is only safe if both partners are free of STI and HIV.

Sex Toys Do not share sex toys! Wash them with soap and water after each use.

Vaginal intercourse It is safe if both partners are free of STI/HIV. The partners should be in a mutually monogamous relationship based on trust. If there is any doubt, use condoms! Remember: No glove? No love! And by the way: The major risk factor for HIV in women is sexual activity with a man.

Anal stimulation, anal intercourse It is safe if both partners are free of STI/HIV and the couple uses lubricant to protect the anal tissue from damage. Wash the penis after anal intercourse, especially before any other sexual activity!

WHAT DOES FREE OF STI/HIV MEAN?
EACH PARTNER SHOULD HAVE TWO NEGATIVE HIV ANTIBODY TESTS AT LEAST SIX MONTHS APART AND EACH PARTNER SHOULD HAVE STI TESTS PERFORMED WITH NEGATIVE RESULTS.

What to do when the test is positive?

Depending on the kind of STI you have your doctor will prescribe treatment and will inform you how to protect yourself and your partner during treatment. Also refer to all the help-line phone numbers in the reference section of this book.

 Are vaccinations available?

No. The only vaccination available is one for hepatitis B. If you get an STI once you can always get it again.

 Will I get cured?

You will have to discuss the infection and the treatment with your doctor. Generally speaking, bacterial infections can be cured quite easily with antibiotics, especially when they are detected early. Viral infections can be treated but not cured. In some cases, like with HPV and herpes you might never get symptoms again after proper treatment, but the virus will stay in your body and you can pass on the virus to a sex partner.

 Is there a sex life after I've been cured from an STI?

Of course! But you might use this experience to protect yourself in the future and practice safer sex! And... there is no excuse because this book tells you how... do it!

Is it possible to have more than one STI at a time?

Yes. Keep in mind: many STIs are easily treated, but all can be dangerous if ignored.

 Do I have to tell my partner?

Yes. Your partner (or your recent partners, if you have had more than one) has to know about your infection so that he/she can go for testing and treatment as well.

 Will my parents find out about the STI testing?

No. Your doctor has to ensure the patient's privacy even if you are under age.

 Can I get infected the first time I have sex?

Yes.

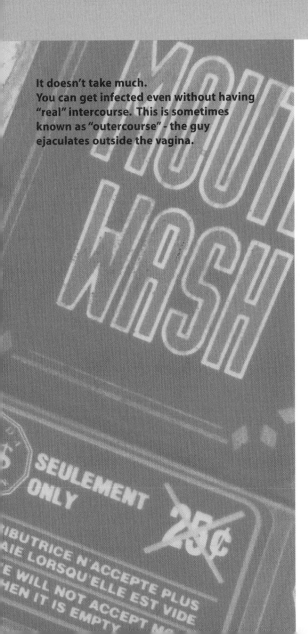

It doesn't take much.
You can get infected even without having "real" intercourse. This is sometimes known as "outercourse" - the guy ejaculates outside the vagina.

Are you at risk of catching an STI or HIV?

We want to help you find out for yourself with a questionnaire. This does not cover all possible situations in which you might be at risk. It should only make you aware that it is extremely likely that you are at risk even if you think you are not! If you answer "YES" to any of the following statements you should make an appointment with your physician and have a test done.

- [ ] My partner has an STI and is currently being treated.
- [ ] My partner has an STI but does not get treatment.
- [ ] I never use condoms.
- [ ] I am in a stable relationship but neither of us has ever had STI testing.
- [ ] I am in a stable relationship but one of us has never had STI testing.
- [ ] I have had a few relationships in the past.
- [ ] I have had no stable relationships but had sex with changing partners.
- [ ] I had an STI before.
- [ ] My partner had an STI before.
- [ ] I or my partner use injection drugs.
- [ ] I had spontaneous sex under the influence of alcohol or drugs.
- [ ] I use condoms sometimes, but not always.

In summary:

Anyone who is involved in any sexual activity, including intercourse, can get infected with an STI. Safer sex reduces this risk. The good news: most STIs can be cured; others can be controlled. The bad news: some, such as HIV, can kill you.

**PROTECT YOURSELF AND YOUR PARTNER BY PRACTICING SAFER SEX.
NO CONDOM? NO SEX.**

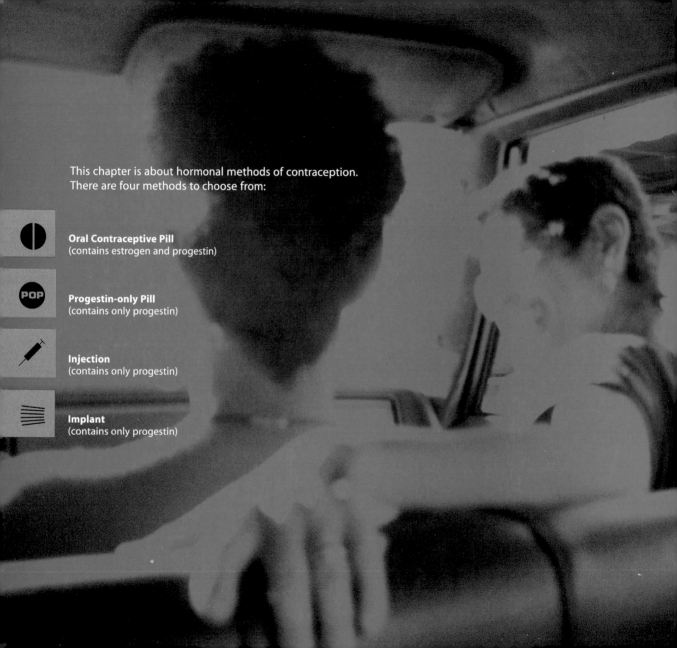

This chapter is about hormonal methods of contraception.
There are four methods to choose from:

Oral Contraceptive Pill
(contains estrogen and progestin)

Progestin-only Pill
(contains only progestin)

Injection
(contains only progestin)

Implant
(contains only progestin)

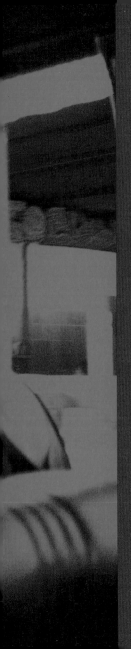

REMOTE CONTROL

THE PILL AND OTHER HORMONAL METHODS

We can compare hormonal contraception to the remote control of a stereo system. The press of a certain button leads to a reaction in your CD player. Hormonal methods work with hormones as "buttons" or couriers, which make certain changes to your system and very effectively prevent the woman from becoming pregnant. For a refresher course on hormones visit The Basics in Chapter 1.

This comparison should not, however, make you believe that you can switch these methods on or off like a CD player! It takes a while for the body to adjust to the hormones. Going on and off the pill for example would unnecessarily put you at risk of becoming pregnant.

Here are the features of this group of methods. They...

- are the most effective reversible contraceptives apart from IUDs.
- require minimal effort and skills in order to be used correctly.
- are independent of intercourse.
- offer many health benefits apart from reliable contraception.
- are designed for long-term use.
- make changes to the systems of your body and may have unwanted effects which normally disappear after the first 1-3 months of use.
- do not protect against STIs and HIV.

COMPARE AND DECIDE:
Hormonal Methods of Contraception

Hormonal methods are the most popular contraceptives in Canada. In the 1998 Canadian Contraception Study, 29% of respondents were using hormonal methods.

	Oral Contraceptive Pill	Progestin-only Pill
Type of drug	tablet to take daily	tablet to take daily
Name	many different brands to choose from	Micronor
Type of hormone	estrogen+progestin	only progestin
Prevents pregnancy primarily by...	stopping ovulation	changing lining of uterus, thickening mucus
Your periods are likely to become...	very regular	somewhat irregular
No bleeding (amenorrhoea) occurs...	very rarely	occasionally
You can stop the method...	any time	any time
You can have a baby afterwards...	wait until you have your regular cycle back (1-3 months usually)	wait until you have your regular cycle back (less than 3 months usually)

Injectable	**Implant**
injection in muscle of upper arm, buttocks or thigh every 10-13 weeks	implant under skin of upper arm every 5 years
Depo-Provera	Norplant
only progestin	only progestin
stopping ovulation	changing lining of uterus, thickening mucus
sparse	somewhat irregular
very often	often
only after the 12- week period is over	any time (appointment for removal necessary!)
wait until you have your regular cycle back (9 months usually)	wait until you have your regular cycle back (1-3 months usually)

The comparison chart will give you a brief overview of hormonal methods. For more details you have to read the individual sections that deal with the methods.

ORAL CONTRACEPTIVE PILL

What is the pill all about?
The pill has to be taken daily whether you have sex or not. It contains two types of hormones (estrogen and progestin). The pill replaces the natural female cycle with an artificial one. The ovaries stop their production and there is no ovulation thus making pregnancy impossible. The pill also changes the mucus in the cervix and the lining of the uterus. This "triple action" makes the pill extremely effective in preventing pregnancy.

What makes the pill so special?
- It is one of the most effective reversible methods of contraception.
- It offers additional health benefits such as more regular cycles, reduced menstrual flow and reduced acne, and it protects against certain cancers.
- It is the most researched method.

Does it protect against sexually transmitted infections and HIV?
No

How effective is the pill in preventing unintended pregnancy?
99.9% effectiveness for the method itself. There is a user failure rate of 3%.

How do I get it?
See a family physician, a gynaecologist or a family planning clinic. A physical exam is recommended but not always necessary and not always performed.

How much does it cost?
Most brands are covered by government health plans. If paid privately: around $20 per month. Check private insurance for reimbursement, dispensing fees in pharmacies. You can also turn to family planning clinics.

Possible problems
There might be some unwanted effects such as bleeding problems (irregular bleeding), breast tenderness, headaches, and nausea. They usually disappear after the first few cycles.

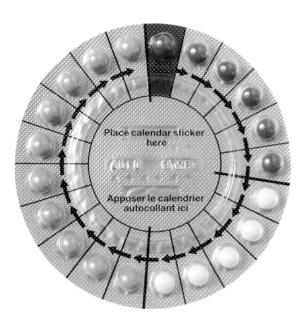

Actual size

WHAT IS THE PILL ALL ABOUT?

The oral contraceptive pill (OC) or simply "the pill" is one of the most researched and the most misunderstood drug in the world. About 100 million women all over the world are relying on it and it is one of the most prescribed medications. The pill is a contraceptive suitable for every healthy woman, regardless of age, that should be used long-term, at least several months in a row. Some women only want to take the pill when they are in a stable relationship and stop taking it when the relationship ends. This is not a good idea. It puts you at risk of unintended pregnancy before you have had enough time to adjust to a new contraceptive method.

There are also many myths and misconceptions surrounding the pill. Please refer to the table on the next page to get an idea about false impressions. You may even believe some of them yourself but let us give you a better picture!

It is widely unknown that the pill offers many health benefits in addition to reliable contraception. Have a look at the table on page 29. We will give you a complete picture of the pill for you to judge, in cooperation with your physician, whether this method is the right choice for you. We want you to be comfortable with your choice. If you have any problems, questions or concerns, discuss them with your health care provider. These people are there for you.

How does the pill work?

Oral contraceptives contain two hormones, a progestin and an estrogen. These hormones, which are similar to the ones produced in your own body, keep the hormone level in your blood above a certain threshold and tell the ovaries not to let any egg cells ripen. In a way, the ovaries are put to rest.

During OC use the lining of the uterus becomes thinner and the entrance to the uterus is blocked by a thicker jelly-like mucus, which makes it more difficult for sperm to move and to reach the uterus. This is called the "triple action of the pill" making it such an effective method of contraception.

MYTH

FACT

MYTHS AND MISCONCEPTIONS

The pill causes cancer

In fact, the pill reduces the risk for certain cancers.

The pill causes weight gain

Some women may experience weight gain, some women weight loss, but weight gain is normally due to an increased appetite and lack of exercise.

The pill causes acne

In fact, most OCs have a favourable effect on acne.

The pill delays future fertility

In fact, most women can get pregnant immediately after stopping the pill. It is a good idea, though, to wait until your natural cycle returns.

All women aged 35 and over must stop taking the pill

Women can take the pill until menopause. You have to stop the pill at age 35 only if you are a smoker.

Women who take the pill should have periodic pill breaks

In fact, once your system is used to the pill you should keep on taking it to avoid irregular cycles and to keep the protection against pregnancy.

It is more risky to take the pill than to be pregnant

In fact, a pregnancy involves a higher risk.

The pill causes birth defects when you become pregnant while taking the pill

This is false.

In the 7-day hormone-free interval, bleeding starts just like in the normal cycle but it is usually less heavy than in women who do not take the pill. Since the pill actually replaces the normal cycle we do not call this a menstruation or period but a withdrawal bleeding. It is caused by the lack of estrogen in the hormone-free interval.

How effective is the pill in preventing unintended pregnancy?

The pill is 99.9% effective, making it the most reliable reversible method of contraception. There is a "user failure rate" of 3%. It is a statistic that reflects that some women make mistakes in taking the pill or that there are certain interactions with other drugs taken at the same time. A little joke on the side: Do you know what the most effective oral contraceptive of them all is? The word NO!

Does the pill protect against sexually transmitted infections and HIV?

No. The pill does not protect against sexually transmitted infections. The simple recipe for safer sex is to go "Dutch treat" or use double protection. Use a condom (male latex condom or female condom) and a spermicide for protection against STIs and take the pill for protection against pregnancy!

How popular is the pill in Canada?

In the 1998 Canadian Contraception Study, the pill was used by 28% of respondents. It is the most popular method of contraception in Canada.

The pill is a good choice for you if you are looking for a method that...

- is simple and very effective.
- makes periods more regular, with less bleeding and less pain.
- you can use from teenage years to menopause.
- allows spontaneity.
- allows you to become pregnant when you stop taking it.
- offers you additional health benefits, known as non-contraceptive benefits.

Look at the table below to get an idea about the motives why Canadian women started taking the pill.

The 1998 Canadian Contraception Study revealed that of all women who chose to take the pill:	
61%	wanted a contraceptive
23%	wanted relief from irregular periods
17%	wanted relief from painful periods
2%	were not satisfied with another method

The pill is not for you, if...

- you have problems with taking the pill daily at the same time, even if you do not have sex.
- you are planning to take it on and off depending on the state of a sexual relationship.
- you have certain health problems that you have to discuss with your doctor (see summary next page).

Where do I get the pill?

You need a prescription first. With the prescription you can go to any pharmacy to get your OCs. To get a prescription you have to go to a family physician, a gynaecologist, public health clinic or to a family planning clinic. You can also contact the health service in your school. Please consider the following:

You're not too crazy about going to a physician for a health exam? Then you might decide to borrow pills from your best girlfriend. Do not even think of it! Your girlfriend's pills were prescribed for her and they might not be good for you!

You are afraid that your parents might find out? If you do not want your parents to know that you are taking the pill you should ask your doctor to keep it secret. The physician will not ask you for permission from your parents to prescribe the pill for you. This is not necessary in Canada. We believe that you are old enough to make responsible decisions about your health.

You are afraid of the exam - the pelvic exam? Do not worry, it is not a big deal. A pelvic exam is not always necessary if you are not sexually active yet. With this exam your doctor wants to make sure that your reproductive organs are healthy.

What to expect on your visit

The first part of your visit consists of questions the doctor will ask you about your health and lifestyle, any previous diseases you may have had, medications you are taking and about your family's health. Some questions might seem a bit too intimate but keep in mind that the physician is on your side. He or she has to know these details about you in order to get a full picture.

If you are already sexually active and you have had intercourse, the physician will then perform a physical exam that includes the following:
- weight and height
- blood pressure
- breast exam
- pelvic exam (Pap smear, STI screen)
- urine and blood sample

The gynaecological exam is performed to make sure that you are not pregnant and that your organs are okay. At the same time you will be tested for any infections. The Pap smear is to find out about cancer cells in your cervix. Don't worry - it is not a big deal.

A first prescription gets you started

You may receive a one-month supply of the pill the physician has chosen for you with a prescription for a 6-12 month period. The physician usually asks you to come back after a few months for a check-up or you may call if you have any side effects or bleeding problems. This second visit is a great chance to ask some more questions or to discuss any unwanted effects. Use this chance to ask anything that came to mind in the past months.

Why are there so many different brands?

A great variety of products allow the health care provider to pick the OC that is right for you. Women have different reactions to hormone content and the type of hormones. Sometimes it might take a while until you find the right brand that suits you best. If acne is a problem you might want to talk to your doctor about OCs that treat acne. Please refer to the summary on page 30.

FOR SOME WOMEN THE PILL IS NOT THE RIGHT CHOICE

➡ You are pregnant.

➡ You suffer from vaginal bleeding other than the normal periods.

➡ You have had blood clots in your legs or elsewhere in your body.

➡ You are a smoker and over 35 years of age.

➡ You have had a stroke, a heart attack or you suffer from chest pain.

➡ You have cancer of the breast or other sex organs or there is a suspicion of a cancer.

➡ You have a liver tumour.

➡ You suffer from liver disease and jaundice.

NON-CONTRACEPTIVE BENEFITS OF ORAL CONTRACEPTIVES

PRESCRIPTIONS

Women who take the pill:

• have less painful periods

• may suffer less from acne

• lose less blood during menstruation and have a lower risk of iron deficiency anaemia

• have a 54% lower risk of ovarian cancer after eight years of taking the pill

• have a 67% lower risk of endometrial cancer after eight years of taking the pill

• have fewer benign ovarian cysts and breast diseases

• have a lower risk of infections in the fallopian tubes and are thus less likely to become infertile

• have fewer bleeding disorders and hot flushes when starting menopause

• are less likely to suffer from tubal (ectopic) pregnancy or to have an abortion

Place calendar sticker here

Apposer le calendrier autocollant ici

And the great thing about it: some of these protective effects continue even after you stop taking the pill.

RAGING HORMONES
Acne and other problems

When there are too many male hormones (androgens) in a woman's body and they are too active, the following problems may show:

- Acne (the oil-producing glands under the skin produce too much oil, the oil gets on the skin surface, bacteria get attached and infections start, which become visible as pimples).
- Oily skin and oily hair (also called seborrhoea).
- Excessive hair growth on the face or on other parts of the body (also called hirsutism).

All brands of combined OCs tend to have a favourable effect on acne. Ask your doctor about a new hormonal treatment that treats severe cases of acne, oily skin and excessive hair growth.

Why are there 21-day and 28-day pill packs?

All OCs available at present are based on a 21-day cycle. Most brands are also available as a 28-day pack. In the 28-day pack there are 21 tablets with hormones and 7 tablets without hormones, called placebos. These pills serve as a reminder to take the pill every day.

Estrogen content can make a difference

The side effects many women are concerned about are often due to the amount of estrogen in the pill. The amount of estrogen in the most recent OCs varies between 20 mcg to 50 mcg depending on the brand. All brands that have 35 mcg or less estrogen content are called low-dose oral contraceptives. Your physician will try to prescribe the pill with the lowest estrogen content for the least amount of side effects. However, side effects normally disappear after the first 1-3 cycles of use. Medical research continues and drug development aims for a smaller hormone content and fewer side effects without, of course, giving up the high reliability of the method.

Can I choose the brand I want?

Apart from clinical arguments there are also certain preferences you as the patient might have. Ask your physician about starter kits from some companies. They contain the product as well as information booklets, and calendars and little pouches to store the pack of tablets in to serve as a reminder to take the pill daily. There are also some interesting gimmicks available (eg. a beeper that reminds you daily).

Issues surrounding the pill

We will address some concerns, which especially come up in discussions with people who are against things that are artificial, such as "artificial hormones" or, let's say, drugs in general. Here is some food for thought:

The pill is not natural It does contain artificial hormones but the hormones used for oral contraceptives are very similar to the ones produced by the body. If natural hormones were used they would still have to be modified in order to be absorbed by the body.

Smoking   Here comes the truth again...smoking is bad for you whether you take the pill or not. Make it your "increase health and save money" resolution and give it up! The risk of heart attack, stroke and blood clots (cardiovascular disease) is increased in women who smoke (in men, too!). However, the risk for these diseases involving the arteries and veins is very low in young women. This changes around age 35. That is the reason why we recommend stopping the pill at the age of 35 if you continue to smoke. Basically the pill makes the dangerous habit of smoking more dangerous. This also applies to nicotine patches or gum used to stop the smoking habit. They contain nicotine as well and they are as bad. Stopping the pill and continuing to smoke over the age of 35 increases the risk of developing heart disease, stroke and cancer.

Cardiovascular disease   This is a general term for diseases of the heart and blood vessels (arteries and veins) such as stroke, heart attack, and thrombosis. There was a big discussion in the early nineties about a certain group of oral contraceptive pills and their effect on the increase of these conditions in users. Armies of specialists have conducted studies and have held lengthy discussions with the following outcome:

- Cardiovascular disease is rare among healthy young women.
- Women at high risk of thrombosis should not take OCs. A risk factor is, for example, a family history of thrombosis.
- Women at high risk of heart attack should not take OCs. Risk factors are severe high blood pressure, family history of heart disease and cigarette smoking after the age of 35.
- Women at high risk of stroke should not use OCs. Risk factors are severe high blood pressure, severe migraines and smoking.

All of this to say that the fear of cardiovascular disease alone should not discourage you from using oral contraceptives. If you have no major risk factors you should not worry. But it is important to talk to your doctor if you have any doubts or fears.

Cancer   Boy, this is a big one! Again there are armies of specialists working on finding out the possible effect of hormones on the development of certain cancers. The same information as in the paragraph on cardiovascular disease applies here. Cancers of the reproductive organs such as cancer of the breast, of the lining of the uterus (endometrium), of the ovaries and of the cervix are very rare among women during their reproductive years. The risk of these cancers rises after menopause.

Breast cancer   Women who do not have children or who have had children very late have a higher risk of developing breast cancer. It is still not clear whether the small increase in breast cancer risk associated with the use of the pill is due to the hormones in the pill itself or whether it is due to the fact that the birth of the first child is delayed by the use of the pill. To make a long story short: you should discuss OC use with your doctor if you have a mother or a sister who developed breast cancer before reaching menopause.

Endometrial cancer   Good news: the chances of getting this kind of cancer, which affects the lining of the uterus are much lower in users of OCs. The incidence of endometrial cancer is reduced by 50 % or more for up to 20 years after OC use. Why? The progestin in the pill reduces the thickness of the lining of the uterus (caused by estrogen) and therefore reduces the risk of endometrial cancer.

Ovarian cancer   More good news: the chances of developing this kind of cancer are 54% lower in women who take the pill for at least 8 years. This protection lasts for many years even after you stop taking the OC. Ovarian cancer risk is linked to the number of cycles of ovulation. Women who do not take OCs and who do not have any children have the highest number of cycles in their lifetime and are at a higher risk of getting this type of cancer. When using an OC the natural cycles are replaced by artificial ones and ovulation does not happen.

Cervical cancer   This cancer is associated with smoking, early age of first intercourse and the number of sexual partners. The Pap smear, which is done during a regular gynaecological exam, is an excellent test for the early detection of this form of cancer.

Lifestyle aspects

Everybody is talking about lifestyle. Why not in the context of contraception?

Here are the features of the pill that might affect your lifestyle:

Determine the time of your periods   If you want to go on a holiday and you do not want to menstruate during this time you can simply skip the hormone-free interval. After you have finished your 21 days of hormone pills you start right away with the next sequence of 21 hormone pills in the next pack.

No more planning ahead   Since you take the pill every day, you are protected against pregnancy every day. You do not have to plan when to have sex or not to have sex. However, for double protection, you should have condoms and a spermicide with you in case your partner does not have any.

Start a daily routine   No benefits without some effort! You have to come up with some sort of routine to remember taking the pill DAILY at a certain time. Keep your pack of tablets by your bed, next to your toothbrush or put it in your wallet to make sure you do not forget to take your pills regularly. Be creative and think of something! When you plan a holiday away from home also remember to take your pills with you. It is difficult to get a replacement when you are in Mexico or on a Caribbean island. The names of brands vary from country to country and you might have to see a physician to get a replacement for your prescription away from home. Have an extra pack with you.

1998 Canadian Contraception Study: THE PILL IN PERSPECTIVE

- Of all Canadian women currently using the pill, 84% had a very favourable opinion of this method.

- Of all Canadian women aged 15-45, 84% have taken the pill at some point in their lives.

- Women's concerns about using the oral contraceptive pill include fear of weight gain (68% of women) and concern about breast cancer (19% of women). Only about one third of women were aware that healthy women can continue to use the pill after the age of 35 and that the pill protects against certain kinds of cancer.

- Only about 15% of women were aware that the health risk related to pregnancy is greater than the risk of taking the pill.

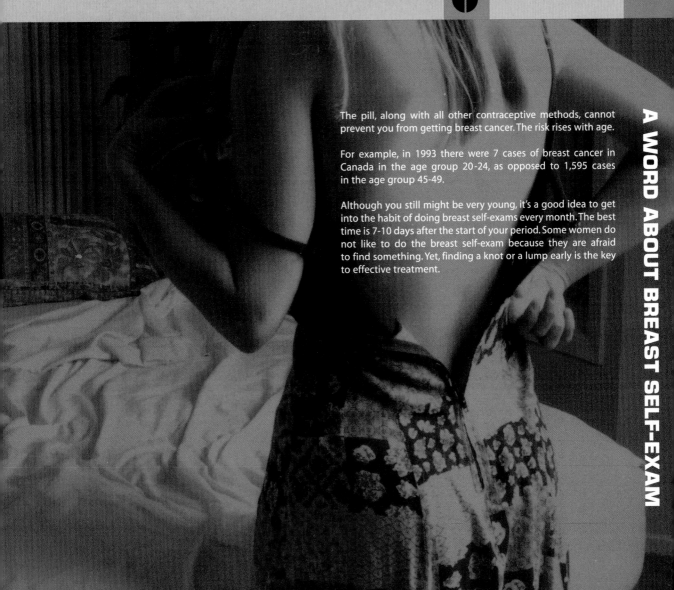

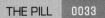
The pill, along with all other contraceptive methods, cannot prevent you from getting breast cancer. The risk rises with age.

For example, in 1993 there were 7 cases of breast cancer in Canada in the age group 20-24, as opposed to 1,595 cases in the age group 45-49.

Although you still might be very young, it's a good idea to get into the habit of doing breast self-exams every month. The best time is 7-10 days after the start of your period. Some women do not like to do the breast self-exam because they are afraid to find something. Yet, finding a knot or a lump early is the key to effective treatment.

A WORD ABOUT BREAST SELF-EXAM

Day 1 start - Day 1 protection.

1. Study the package insert. It sounds like a boring idea but the package inserts of OCs are usually well done. They tell you a great deal about the pill you chose.

   We recommend the "Day 1 start." Start the pack on the first day of a menstrual period. Some package inserts recommend other start days. These other start days affect the recommendations for missed pills. That's why it is so important to read the package insert.

2. Make use of the stickers and other support tools such as special packaging to help you remember to take the pill regularly.

3. Make an appointment with your doctor immediately if certain problems occur. Like any other medication, side effects can occur which need immediate attention. In your package insert you can read about these warning signs.

How do I get the routine, how to remember?

As a new starter you should choose the Day 1 start.

When you start taking the pill on Day 1 of your cycle (first day of your period) you enjoy protection against pregnancy from Day 1.

The first tablet in every pack that follows will always be taken on the same day of the week. If you start taking the pill on a later day in the cycle you have to use a backup method of contraception for the first 21 days.

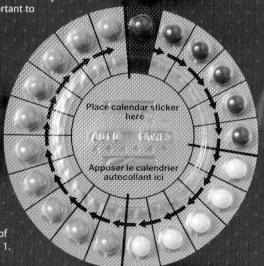

Place calendar sticker here

Apposer le calendrier autocollant ici

Here is how you take the pill:

Monophasic 21-day pack:
In a 21-day pack all pills contain hormones. Take the first pill of the pack on Day 1 of your cycle, which is the first day of your period. Take one pill every day until the pack is finished. Then wait 7 days and start the next pack. During the 7-day hormone-free interval you will experience bleeding. However, it is very important that you start your new pack after 7 days regardless of whether bleeding has occurred or not, or whether it is still going on.

Monophasic 28-day pack:
In a 28-day pack only the first 21 pills contain hormones. Different colours indicate the two types of pills. Take the first pill of the pack on Day 1 of your cycle, which is the first day of your period.

Take one pill every day until the pack is finished. Then start with a new pack. From day 22-28 you will experience bleeding.

Biphasic / Triphasic pills:
Follow the same schedule as with the monophasic preparations. Different colours indicate the different hormone content in the tablets.

TROUBLESHOOTING

The following are very rare warning signs that should signal you to stop taking the pill and to go directly to the emergency room of a hospital near you:

Strong pain in the chest or in the legs, severe pain in the abdomen, shortness of breath, sudden loss of vision or disturbance of vision, severe headaches or yellowing of the skin are warning signs that there is something wrong with you.

Here are other signs that are much less serious and do not warrant stopping the pill before talking to your physician. These signs are not hazardous to your health and normally disappear after the first 1-3 cycles of taking the pill. They also do not impair the effectiveness of your OC unless you stop taking it regularly.

Never stop taking the pill without talking to your doctor first.

Breakthrough bleeding

Bleeding which occurs during the 21 days of pill taking. It can be real bleeding or just spotting. The likelihood of breakthrough bleeding is higher during the first 3 cycles of OC use. The body needs to adapt to these new kinds of hormones and it takes a while. Many studies have been conducted but no single brand of OCs has really proven itself to be the best in preventing unscheduled bleeding. Use the brand for at least 3-4 cycles. If the problem does not stop, keep on taking the pill and consult your physician again.

No bleeding at all (amenorrhoea)

It occurs in 5-10% of cycles. This is nothing to worry about unless you forgot to take the pill or the pill was not absorbed by your body (due to vomiting for example) and you had unprotected intercourse. In this case no bleeding can mean that you are pregnant!

Mood changes

In most cases irritability or depressed mood has other causes than the use of an OC.

Weight gain

Studies comparing OCs with other methods of contraception failed to show any significant weight gain in OC users. With the use of low-dose pills (35mcg of estrogen content or less), weight gain is minimal and is often due to normal age related weight gain. It is possible that during the first months of use an increased appetite may lead to eating more. Keep that in mind and beware!

Acne

Combined OCs usually have a favourable effect on acne. If acne is a big problem for you, ask your doctor about a new hormonal treatment.

Chloasma

Chloasma are brown spots on the face, which develop in some women as a response to estrogen. This is an overproduction of pigments. The use of a sunscreen prevents the development of chloasma because it is a response to sun exposure just like tanning. You might have to see a dermatologist if it does not get better.

Nausea

This is common during the first three cycles of OC use. Taking the pill at bedtime or together with food might help.

Vomiting and diarrhoea

This might make the pill less effective. You should use a backup method of contraception such as the condom.

Pregnancy

If you become pregnant while taking an OC you should stop taking the pill immediately. But there is no reason for panic because there is no increased risk of birth defects as a result of OC use during pregnancy.

Headaches

Headaches which occur after starting a pill may be a reason to stop taking it. Consult your physician first! Women who experience headaches during the hormone-free interval can overcome this problem by taking their OC continuously.

Problem with vision

If you wear contact lenses you may experience some discomfort or change of vision. If this persists you should contact your optometrist for refitting.

Breast tenderness

Usually nothing to worry about.

Drug interactions

Always inform your physician about all the drugs you are taking. They might change the action of your birth control pill. Some medications such as certain antibiotics can cause the failure of your OCs in preventing pregnancy. On the other hand your pill might cause other medications you were prescribed to fail as well. It is important to talk to your health care provider and/or your pharmacist about it. If you have to take a medication which makes the pill less effective, always use another method as a backup.

Troubleshooting cont'd ▸▸

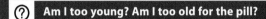

⑦ Am I too young? Am I too old for the pill?

There is no lower age limit because of the many benefits of the pill, which by far outweigh the risks of an unintended pregnancy. You do not even have to wait until you want to have sex. After you have your first menstrual bleeding, the pill can help regulate your cycles and can lessen the pain during your menstruation. You are also not too old. The recommendation that women should stop taking OCs when they are past 35 is history. Women who do not smoke can take the pill up to menopause.

⑦ Should I interrupt taking the pill every once in a while?

Absolutely not. There shouldn't be any interruptions unless you WANT to get pregnant.

⑦ Will the doctor tell my parents?

No. Physicians must respect confidentiality.

⑦ When taking a 21-day pill, can I have sex during the hormone-free interval?

Yes, you are protected all the time, provided you have been taking your tablets regularly.

⑦ Will I be able to become pregnant after stopping the pill?

Yes, no problem. After stopping the pill you should wait and use other methods of contraception until your natural cycle is back to normal. This makes it easier to calculate the beginning of a pregnancy.

TROUBLESHOOTING

❓ What do I do when my pill gets bad media?

The OC is the most researched medication that exists. No wonder! It is taken by more than 100 million women across all continents. Because there are so many people still researching and so many women who rely on this type of contraception, media around the world is always very interested in new stories about the pill. If you ever read or hear something scary about the oral contraceptive do not panic. Continue taking your OC daily and make an appointment to see your doctor who can explain what the problem is all about. Do not stop taking it and risk a pregnancy!

Here is some good news that was in the media lately:

January 1999: A study in the prestigious British Medical Journal confirmed that there are no negative long-term effects due to the use of OCs. After 10 years of stopping the pill the risk of getting cancer or a stroke is the same in women who took the pill as compared to women who never took it.

June 1999: Japan has finally approved the use of the pill. It was one of the only countries in the world left where women did not have access to this simple, safe and effective method of birth control.

June 1999: A study published in the British Medical Journal found no increased risk of heart attacks in women who are taking the pill.

Missed pills ⚠

No panic! You will have to use a backup method. Missing tablets at the beginning or end of the 21-day cycle has the effect of lengthening the hormone-free interval. If the hormone-free interval exceeds seven days, the risk of ovulation and possible pregnancy increases. Forgetting tablets in the second or third week of the 21-day cycle may also increase the risk of ovulation.

INSTRUCTIONS REGARDING MISSED PILLS (FOR THE DAY 1 START):

▶ If one pill is missed, you should take it as soon as you remember. This may mean taking two pills in one day.

▶ If you miss two pills in a row during Week 1 and 2 of the pack, you should take two pills on the day you remember and two on the following day. You should use a backup method of contraception until you have taken seven hormone pills in a row.

▶ If you miss two pills in a row in Week 3 of the pack, throw out the remainder of the pack and start a new pack on the day you remember. You may not have a period this month.

▶ If you miss three pills in a row, throw out the remainder of the pack and start a new pack on the day you remember. You should use a backup method such as the sponge and the condom if you have intercourse in the first seven days of the new pack. You may not have a period this month.

▶ If you miss 2 menstrual periods in a row, take a pregnancy test.

PROGESTIN-ONLY PILL [POP]

What is the POP all about?

The POP contains one hormone, a progestin. It interferes with the natural cycle. The ovaries keep working. The progestin acts on the lining of the uterus walls and on the jelly-like mucus at the entrance of the cervix to make it difficult for sperm to get through. The POP also inhibits ovulation in 60% of users.

What makes the method so special?

- It is one of the most effective reversible methods of contraception.
- It can be used by many women who are otherwise not allowed to use the pill because of certain health problems.
- It offers additional health benefits such as reduced menstrual pain and menstrual blood flow and protection against certain cancers.

Does it protect against sexually transmitted infections and HIV?

No

How effective is the POP in preventing unintended pregnancy?

90-99%

How do I get it?

See a family physician, a gynaecologist or family planning clinic and ask about Micronor. Start the first day of your period and take one tablet every day at the same time until the pack is empty. Then start the next pack.

- There is no hormone-free interval.
- You have to use a backup method during the first month of taking the POP.

How much does it cost?

Approximately $20 per month. Check private insurance for reimbursement, dispensing fees in pharmacies. You can also turn to family planning clinics.

Possible problems

- Forgetting pills. This method is not very forgiving if you forget to take the pills regularly.
- Irregular bleeding.

The POP offers some health benefits apart from reliable contraception. These "non-contraceptive" benefits apply to all progestin-only methods.

Non-contraceptive benefits of progestin-only pill, injection and implant:

- Reduces the risk of cancer of the endometrium and ovaries.
- Reduces risk of inflammation in the fallopian tubes and prevents infertility.
- Reduces menstrual pain, pre-menstrual pain, pain associated with endometriosis and chronic pain.
- Possibly reduces frequency of seizures.

How does the POP work?

The hormone progestin in the POP sends certain messages to the brain and to the sex organs to change the lining of the uterus. This lining, the endometrium, becomes unfriendly for an egg to settle in and develop. It also changes the jelly-like mucus at the entrance of the cervix. This mucus becomes thicker and more difficult for the sperm to go through. Unlike the oral contraceptive pill (OC), the POP does not fully prevent ovulation. In 40% of all cycles ovulation will still occur.

How effective is the POP in preventing unintended pregnancy?

This method is 90-99% effective. It is as effective as the OC if taken correctly, meaning absolutely regularly, at the same time of day, every day!

Does the POP protect against sexually transmitted infections and HIV?

No. The POP does not protect you and your partner from STIs. The simple recipe for safer sex is to go "Dutch treat" or use double protection! Use a condom (male latex condom or female condom) for protection against STIs and get the POP for protection against pregnancy!

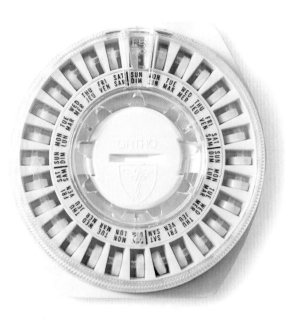

Actual size

WHAT IS THE POP ALL ABOUT?

The progestin-only pill is a birth control pill, which contains only one synthetic hormone: progestin. This method is only for women who can remember to take a tablet every day at the same time. This method allows for no error in pill taking because it contains only one hormone and can only prevent unintended pregnancy when taken absolutely regularly. It is a good choice for women who are breast-feeding. There is only one brand available in Canada, which is called Micronor. It contains 35 mcg of norethindrone.

You will receive a prescription for roughly one year. The physician might ask you to come back after three months for a check-up. This second visit is a great chance to ask some more questions or to discuss any unwanted effects. Use this chance to ask anything that came to mind in the past three months.

How do I take my POP, how do I remember?

1 Study the package insert. It sounds like a boring idea but the package inserts of contraceptives are the best package inserts available. It tells you a great deal about the POP.

2 Make yourself familiar with the dial pack.

3 Call your doctor immediately if certain problems occur. As with any other medication, side effects can occur which need immediate attention. In your package insert you can read about these warning signs.

Use the Day 1 start.

As a new starter you should choose the "Day 1 start." On the first day of your cycle, which is the first day of bleeding, you take the first pill in the pack. After that you continue to take one pill every day until the pack is finished. Then you immediately start the next pack. With the POP there is no hormone-free interval like with the oral contraceptive. Make it a daily routine to take one pill every day at the same time. This method only allows for a maximum delay of three hours. During the first month, you have to use a backup method.

The POP is a good choice for you, if you are looking for a method that:

- is very reliable.
- has no estrogen-related side effects.
- makes your periods lighter.
- you can stop any time if you want to have a baby.
- offers certain additional health benefits.
- is a good alternative for women
  - who are over the age of 35 and still smoke.
  - who suffer from migraine headaches.
  - who are breast-feeding.
  - who suffer from sickle cell anaemia.

Basically, the POP is an option for every woman seeking effective contraception.

The POP is not for you, if you:

- cannot remember to take a pill every day at the same time.
- cannot tolerate bleeding irregularities.
- develop cysts on the ovaries.
- are already pregnant.
- suffer from vaginal bleeding other than your period.

Where do I get the POP?

You need to make an appointment with your family physician, a gynaecologist or at a family planning clinic. The interview and the health check-up are the same as with the pill. Please refer to pages 27-28.

Issues surrounding the POP

Breast-feeding / after delivery of a baby The POP can be taken right after the delivery of a baby. If the woman chooses to breast-feed, the POP will not have any effect on the quality or quantity of the breast milk.

Cardiovascular disease The use of the POP does not increase the risk of cardiovascular disease. In fact, women with a history of cardiovascular disease are encouraged to choose the POP as a safe contraceptive method.

TROUBLESHOOTING

Here are some unwanted effects that cause women to stop taking progestin-only pills because they do not know that these effects normally end within three months of use. We advise you not to stop taking the POP before you talk to your physician about the problems.

Missed pills

If a pill is forgotten or vomited, a backup method must be used for at least 7 days.

Unscheduled bleeding

The likelihood of unscheduled bleeding is higher in the first three months of the use of the POP. You might find your cycle a little mixed up. The body needs to adapt to this new kind of hormone and it takes a while.

No bleeding at all (amenorrhoea)

This is possible with the use of the POP. This is nothing to worry about unless you forgot to take the pill or the pill did not get absorbed by the body (due to vomiting, flu-like illness, diarrhoea, drug interaction) and you had unprotected intercourse. In this case no bleeding can mean that you are pregnant!

Nausea

This is uncommon with this kind of pill. Taking the POP at bedtime or together with food might help.

Vomiting

Vomiting might make the pill less effective. You should use a backup method of contraception such as the condom for 7 days.

Pregnancy

If you become pregnant while taking the POP you should stop taking it immediately. But there is no reason for panic because there is no increased risk of birth defects as a result of POP use during pregnancy.

Drug interactions

Always inform your physician about all the drugs you are taking. They might change the action of your POP. Some medications can cause the failure of your pill in preventing pregnancy. On the other hand your POP might cause other medications you were prescribed to fail as well. It is important to talk to your health care provider and/or your pharmacist about it.

IMPORTANT

During the first month you have to use a backup method of contraception such as the male latex condom or the female condom because the POP takes a while to become fully effective in preventing pregnancy.

INJECTION

What is the injection contraceptive all about?
It contains one hormone, a progestin. It interferes with the natural cycle, but does not completely replace it like the oral contraceptive pill does. It stops ovulation and acts on the lining of the uterus walls and on the jelly-like mucus at the entrance of the cervix to make it difficult for sperm to get through.

What makes the method so special?
- It is one of the most effective reversible methods of contraception.
- It is a "no-worry" method because you do not have to follow a daily pill-taking routine.
- It can be used by women who cannot take estrogen due to certain health conditions.
- It provides contraception for 12 weeks.
- It offers additional health benefits.

How effective is the injection in preventing unintended pregnancy?
99.7% effective. The failure rate is 3 pregnancies in 1000 women who used the method for 1 year.

Does it protect against sexually transmitted infections and HIV?
No

How do I get it?
See a family physician, a gynaecologist or family planning clinic and ask about Depo-Provera. You should get your first injection during the first 5 days of your menstrual cycle. This provides effective contraception for 12 weeks. Depo-Provera starts to be effective 24 hours after its injection. After 10-13 weeks you have to go back for a renewal injection.

How much does it cost?
Check reimbursement, if private: around $35 per injection. You can also turn to family planning clinics.

Possible problems
Bleeding irregularities and weight gain are possible concerns with this method. 50% of women stop their periods altogether within one year of use.

WHAT IS THE INJECTION CONTRACEPTIVE ALL ABOUT?

The injection contraceptive is like a vaccine. It has to be renewed every 10-13 weeks (four times a year). It contains only one synthetic hormone. It is a new contraceptive method that is available in Canada since 1997 under the name Depo-Provera.

The injection offers additional health benefits, known as "non-contraceptive benefits", which are the same for all progestin-only methods of contraception. Please refer to page 41.

How does the injection contraceptive work?

The hormone progestin (medroxyprogesterone acetate) sends certain messages to the brain and to the sex organs to stop the monthly release of an egg (ovulation). The endometrium becomes unfriendly for an egg to settle in and develop if ovulation occurs. It also changes the jelly-like mucus at the entrance of the cervix. This mucus becomes thicker and makes it more difficult for sperm to move and travel to the uterus.

How effective is the injection in preventing unintended pregnancy?

This method is 99.7% effective. In other words: In 1000 women who used the method for 1 year only 3 pregnancies were reported. This method is the second most effective reversible method of contraception.

Does the injection protect against sexually transmitted infections and HIV?

No. The injection does not protect you and your partner from STIs. The simple recipe for safer sex is to go "Dutch treat" and use double protection! Use a condom (male latex condom or female condom) and a spermicide for protection against STIs and get the 10-13 week injection for protection against pregnancy!

How popular is the injection in Canada?

In the 1998 Canadian Contraception Study the injection was used by 1% of all respondents. It is a new method that was approved as a contraceptive in Canada in 1997.

The injection contraceptive is a good choice for you, if you are looking for a method that:

- is simple and very effective.
- requires no day-to-day routine.
- has no estrogen-related side effects.
- is long-lasting (10-13 weeks).
- makes your periods lighter; in 50% of women the periods will stop within one year of use.
- offers certain additional health benefits.
- is a good alternative for women
  - who cannot take an oral contraceptive pill due to the estrogen.
  - who have a problem with taking the pill or the progestin-only pill on a daily basis.
  - who are over the age of 35 and still smoke.
  - who suffer from migraine headaches.
  - who are breast-feeding.
  - who suffer from sickle cell anaemia.

Basically, the injection is an option for every woman seeking effective contraception. However,

The injection is not for you, if you:

- cannot tolerate bleeding irregularities.
- are afraid of any weight gain due to increased appetite.
- cannot take regular appointments every 90 days for the renewal of the injection.
- want to get pregnant fast after stopping the injections.
- are already pregnant.
- suffer from vaginal bleeding other than your period.

HOW DO I GET STARTED?

Try to time your visit

Try to time your visit so that you can get the injection during the first five days of your menstrual cycle, meaning during the first few days of bleeding. Depo-Provera is fully effective in preventing pregnancy 24 hours after its injection. No backup method is required.

Problem with the right timing?

If you do not or cannot (example: you have no periods for a while) receive Depo-Provera during the first 5 days of a normal menstrual period, you should have a pregnancy test before the injection to ensure that you are not pregnant. If the test is negative and you get the injection, you should use another contraceptive method as a backup for a period of 3-4 weeks following the injection.

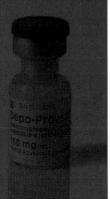

Where do I get the injection?

You need to make an appointment with your family physician, a gynaecologist or at a family planning clinic. The interview and the health check-up are the same as with the pill. Please refer to pages 27-28.

What to expect during the procedure.

You get an injection into a muscle in the upper arm, buttocks or thigh. A nurse normally does this. Immediately make an appointment for your next visit in 10-13 weeks. That way you will not forget!

Issues surrounding the injection contraceptive

Breast-feeding / after delivery of a baby If the woman wants to breast-feed she should wait until at least 3 days after delivery before having the injection. The progestin has no effect on the quality and quantity of breast milk. If she does not want to breast-feed, the injection can be done right after the delivery of the baby.

Cardiovascular disease The injection contraceptive does not increase the risk of cardiovascular disease. In fact, the injection may be an appropriate contraceptive for women with a history of cardiovascular disease. They are encouraged to choose the injection as a safe contraceptive method.

Return to fertility With the injection the return to fertility takes longer than with the oral contraceptive pill. Once you have had the injection it will take 12 weeks for your body to work off the injected hormones. After this period it will take an average of nine months to ovulate and return to your natural cycle again. Studies have shown the following results: at 6 months following the last injection, 52% of women who wanted to become pregnant became pregnant, at 1 year, 76%, and at 2 years, 92%.

TROUBLESHOOTING

Here are some unwanted effects, which cause concern in women and make them uncomfortable with this method. These effects normally stop after the first few months of use.

Unscheduled bleeding or no bleeding

This is one of the big concerns in women using the injection. Many women will experience unpredictable bleeding or spotting following the first two injections (6 months). Some women stop bleeding altogether within the first year of use. If you experience some bleeding problems do not hesitate to talk to your doctor about it. There are several ways to treat this problem.

Weight gain

This is due to increased appetite caused by the progestin in the injection and it happens to about 50% of women. Those women who gained weight, gained approximately 2.5kg in the first year of use, 3.7kg after the second year, and 6.3 kg after the fourth year. If you gain weight, rule out other causes such as change in diet, lack of physical activity or other medications, and maintain good eating habits and regular exercise.

FOR MORE INFORMATION:
call **1-888-671-3376**
or visit the website: **www.birthcontrol.pnu.ca**

Decreased bone density

This effect is not proven. If it occurs, it can be reversed after stopping injections. You should discuss this with your physician to find out whether this could be a problem for you.

Drug interactions

Always inform your physician about all the drugs you are taking.

Late for the next appointment

The injection of progestin is a reliable contraceptive for 10-13 weeks. If you cannot make it to the next appointment on time to get your new injection you have to use a back-up method of contraception such as the condom (male or female condom). Upon your next visit your doctor or the nurse will have to do a pregnancy test to make sure you are not pregnant before giving you the next injection. The company that produces Depo-Provera offers a cost-free reminder service. You will find more details in the patient information that you will receive when getting your first injection.

IMPLANT

What is the implant all about?
Norplant contains one hormone, a progestin. It stops ovulation and acts on the lining of the uterus walls and on the jelly-like mucus at the entrance of the cervix to make it difficult for sperm to get through.

What makes the method so special?
- It is the most effective reversible method of contraception.
- It is a "no-worry" method because you do not have to follow a daily pill-taking routine.
- It can be used by women who cannot take estrogen.
- It provides contraception for 5 years.
- It offers additional health benefits.

Does it protect against sexually transmitted infections and HIV?
No

How effective is the implant in preventing unintended pregnancy?
99.8% effective. The failure rate is 2 pregnancies in 1000 women who used the method for 1 year.

How do I get it?
See a family physician, a gynaecologist or family planning clinic and ask about Norplant. A small surgical procedure under local anaesthesia is necessary to place the six match-size rods under the skin of your arm.

How much does it cost?
Check reimbursement, if private: around $450. You can also turn to family planning clinics.

Possible problems
Bleeding irregularities, weight gain. But, these problems are less frequent with the implant than they are with the injection!

WHAT IS THE IMPLANT ALL ABOUT?

The implant, available in Canada under the name Norplant, consists of six match-sized plastic strips, which are inserted beneath the skin under your arm. The strips are 34 mm long, and 2.4 mm in diameter. The strips release a constant dose of the progestin levonorgestrel, which provides very effective contraception for a period of 5 years.

The implant offers additional health benefits, known as "non-contraceptive benefits", which are the same for all progestin-only methods of contraception. Please refer to page 41.

How does the implant work?

The hormone progestin (levonorgestrel) in the implant sends certain messages to the brain and to the sex organs to change the lining of the uterus. The lining, the endometrium, becomes unfriendly for an egg to settle in and develop. It also changes the jelly-like mucus at the entrance of the cervix. This mucus becomes thicker and more difficult for the sperm to go through. The implant may also prevent ovulation, especially in the first two years of use.

How effective is the implant in preventing unintended pregnancy?

This method is the most effective reversible method of contraception. It is 99.8% effective. In other words: in 1000 women who used the method for one year, 2 pregnancies were reported. There is practically no user failure possible.

Does the implant protect against sexually transmitted infections and HIV?

No. The implant does not protect you and your partner from STIs. The simple recipe for safer sex is to go "Dutch treat" and use double protection! Use a condom (male latex condom or female condom) and a spermicide for protection against STIs and get the implant for protection against pregnancy!

The implant is a good choice for you if you are looking for a method that:

- is simple and very effective.
- requires no day-to-day routine.
- has no estrogen-related side effects.
- has a very long-lasting effect (5 years).
- makes your periods lighter or even disappear.
- offers certain additional health benefits.
- is a good alternative for women
  - who cannot take the oral contraceptive pill due to the estrogen.
  - who have a problem with taking the pill or the progestin-only pill on a daily basis.

Basically, the implant is an option for every woman seeking effective, very long-term contraception.

The implant is not for you, if you:

- cannot tolerate bleeding irregularities.
- are afraid of any weight gain due to increased appetite.
- are afraid of the possible development of cysts on the ovaries.
- are afraid of even small surgical procedures (this is necessary for insertion and removal of implant).
- are already pregnant.
- suffer from vaginal bleeding other than your normal periods.

The 1998 Canadian Contraception Study revealed that:

1%	of respondents in the study use Norplant

HOW DO I GET STARTED?

You have to time your visit so that the insertion of Norplant can be done during the first few days of your menstrual cycle, during the first few days of bleeding. Norplant is fully effective in preventing pregnancy twenty-four hours after its insertion. No backup method is required.

Where do I get the implant?

You need to make an appointment with your family physician, a gynaecologist or a family planning clinic. The interview and the health check-up are the same as with the pill. Please refer to page 27-28.

What to expect during the procedure.

The best place for the six strips is under the upper inner arm. The doctor or nurse will give you a local anaesthetic to prevent you from having pain. A small cut will open the skin. After the cut, the skin will be lifted and the six strips are placed under it. In most cases they will not show through the skin. Local inflammation and infections at the site of the implant are very rare.

Issues surrounding the implant

Breast-feeding / after delivery of a baby If the woman wants to breast-feed she should wait until she is well established in her breast-feeding before having the implant inserted.

If she does not want to breast-feed the insertion can be done right after the delivery of the baby.

Cardiovascular disease The implant does not increase the risk of cardiovascular disease. In fact, women with a history of cardiovascular disease are encouraged to choose implants as a safe contraceptive method.

Return to fertility If you wish to become pregnant you can ask your physician to remove the implants at any time. On average it takes a woman 1-3 months to resume her normal cycle following the removal of the implant, enabling her to become pregnant.

TROUBLESHOOTING

Here are some unwanted effects that cause women to worry because they do not know that these effects normally end within three months of use.

Headache

Rare, but if persistent, contact your doctor.

Unscheduled bleeding or no bleeding

This is the most common side effect with the implant. If you experience some bleeding problems do not hesitate to talk to your doctor about it. There is a way to treat the problem without removing the implant and losing the contraceptive protection of Norplant. It is also possible that the periods stop altogether. This is nothing to worry about because the possibility that you will become pregnant with Norplant is extremely low. 12% of women experience this problem (amenorrhoea) with the implant.

Weight gain

Over five years of use, Norplant users gain an average of 2.5 kg. This differs from individual to individual. Usually the weight gain is due to an increased appetite. Watching what and how much you eat plus regular exercise can help solve this problem!

Drug interactions

Always inform your physician about all the drugs you are taking.

Other effects

Depression, ovarian cysts, breast tenderness and acne have been reported, but they are very rare.

This chapter is about the following methods:

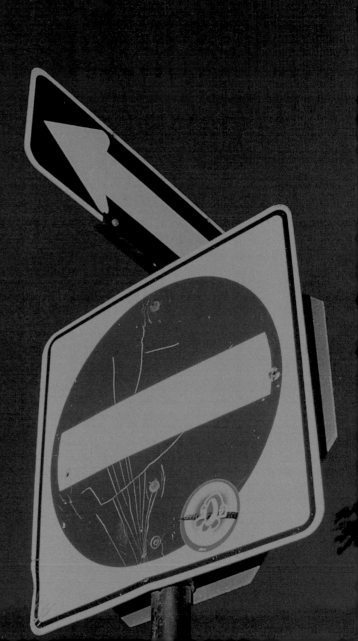

Condom

Female Condom

Contraceptive Sponge

Lea Contraceptive

Diaphragm

Cervical Cap

Spermicides

For your own and your partner's health:
Say NO to sex if your partner says NO to condoms.
No glove, no love!

BARRIER METHODS

KEYS TO SAFER SEX

The biggest advantage of barrier methods is their role in the prevention of sexually transmitted infections. The female and male latex condoms are the best performers when it comes to STI and HIV protection. They are the only available contraceptives that offer very good protection against these infections. As you will find out by reading this chapter, other barrier methods offer some protection against STIs as well.

Here are some additional features of barrier methods:
- Barrier methods do not prevent pregnancy as effectively as hormonal or surgical methods, but they can be used in combination to practice safer sex for double protection. Combinations could be:
  - Pill and condom
  - IUD and condom
  - Sponge and male condom
  - Male condom and spermicide

- Barrier methods are very convenient: no doctor's appointment needed (except for the fitting of a diaphragm or cap) and you only use the method when you have sex.
- Barrier methods target sperm: one way to target sperm is to create a barrier so that male sperm cannot reach the cervix, uterus and then the fallopian tubes where there might be an egg waiting to be fertilized. The other way is to destroy sperm upon contact, which is done by spermicides or the sponge. The sponge is impregnated with spermicides.
- Barrier methods have no systemic effects on your body: they do not interfere with how your body functions.
- Barrier methods require practice to use them correctly each time you have intercourse.

In the 1998 Canadian Contraception Study, 26% of the respondents were using barrier methods of contraception. The following table gives you a summary of the most popular barrier methods. *

COMPARE AND DECIDE :
Barrier Methods of Contraception

	Condom	Female condom
Nature of the method	barrier	barrier
Physician appointment necessary	no	no
Spermicide needed at time of insertion	recommended	no
Additional spermicide needed for each new act of intercourse	recommended	no
Can be used during menstruation	yes	yes
When to insert/apply	rolled over erect penis before intercourse	anytime before intercourse
When to remove	after ejaculation	after intercourse and before standing up
SAFETY: **Maximum time device can be left in place**	no time restrictions	8 hours
The device is good for	only 1 application	only 1 application
If lubricant is desired	only water-based	water or oil-based

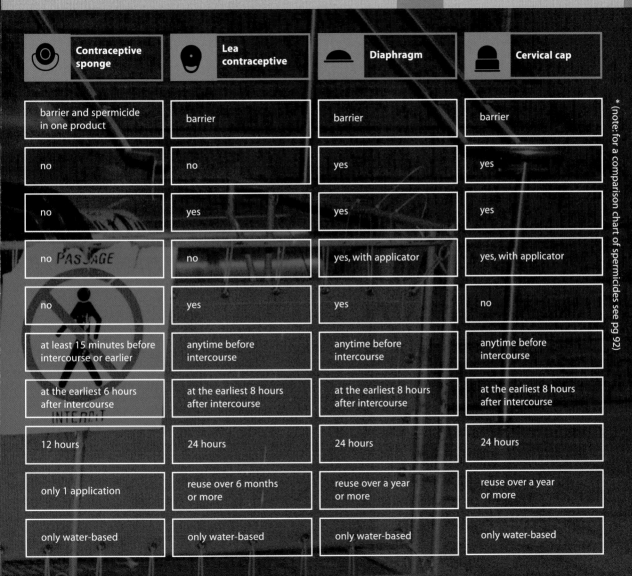 **Contraceptive sponge**	**Lea contraceptive**	**Diaphragm**	**Cervical cap**
barrier and spermicide in one product	barrier	barrier	barrier
no	no	yes	yes
no	yes	yes	yes
no	no	yes, with applicator	yes, with applicator
no	yes	yes	no
at least 15 minutes before intercourse or earlier	anytime before intercourse	anytime before intercourse	anytime before intercourse
at the earliest 6 hours after intercourse	at the earliest 8 hours after intercourse	at the earliest 8 hours after intercourse	at the earliest 8 hours after intercourse
12 hours	24 hours	24 hours	24 hours
only 1 application	reuse over 6 months or more	reuse over a year or more	reuse over a year or more
only water-based	only water-based	only water-based	only water-based

* (note: for a comparison chart of spermicides see pg 92)

CONDOM

What is the condom all about?
A latex or sheep membrane sheath which is rolled over the penis. The condom acts as a barrier. It prevents the exchange of body fluids and semen. The latex condom protects against most STIs and HIV and against pregnancy. The sheep membrane condom protects only against pregnancy. The condom should be used in combination with a spermicide.

What makes the condom so special?
- The condom has benefits other than protection against pregnancy: latex condoms protect against most STIs and HIV, cervical cancer and infertility.
- It can be used in combination with other methods to practice safer sex and to get double protection.
- All condoms can become part of the sex play and can improve sexual relations.

Does the condom protect against sexually transmitted infections and HIV?
Yes, but not 100%. Latex condoms protect against STIs and HIV with the exception of herpes and HPV. Sheep membrane condoms do not protect against STIs and HIV.

How effective is the condom in preventing unintended pregnancy?
Used perfectly the probability of failure during the first year of use is 3 %.
The typical use failure rate is higher: 12%.

How do I get it?
Prescription-free in vending machines, drugstores, condom shops, on-line.

How do I use it?
You roll it on the erect penis before intercourse.

If you use a lubricant
Only water-based lubricants.

How much does it cost?
Fifty cents and up per condom.

Possible problems
- Application problems, lack of practice.
- Some couples complain about a lack of sensitivity.
- Condom breakage due to rough handling, use of oil-based lubricant and passed expiry date.
- Latex allergy.

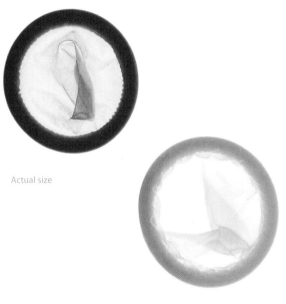

Actual size

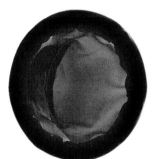

WHAT IS THE CONDOM ALL ABOUT?

Condoms are sheaths made out of rubber (latex) or animal material (sheep membrane), which are placed on the erect penis. Condoms are the only method of contraception that provides protection against pregnancy and STIs including HIV.

People with a latex allergy can use sheep membrane condoms. Sheep membrane condoms protect only against unintended pregnancy and not against STIs and HIV. Viruses and bacteria are so small that they can pass through the pores of these condoms.

Soon there will be a new type of condom on the Canadian market that is made of the same material as the female condom (polyurethane). This offers the same protection as the latex condom, is stronger and cannot cause latex allergies.

Condoms also offer protection from infections for same sex couples. Condoms are highly recommended for sex practices such as oral and anal sex.

Since no other method of birth control (except the female condom) offers a nearly full protection against infections like the latex condom does, the latex condom is a great protector that should be used in combination with other methods of contraception to practice safer sex.

The latex condom protects against:

- HIV.
- STIs (except HPV and herpes).
- Pregnancy.
- Ectopic pregnancy.
- Lower tract infections (vaginitis).
- Upper tract infections (pelvic inflammatory disease).
- Infections that can harm the fetus during pregnancy and childbearing.
- Blocked fallopian tubes, which cause infertility.
- Cancer of the genitals.

How does the condom work?

Condoms act as a barrier and are protective in many ways. Latex condoms **protect the man** from coming into contact with secretions from the vagina, wounds inside the vagina or menstrual blood and prevent him from catching an infection. Latex condoms **protect the woman** from contact with semen thus protecting her from unintended pregnancy. At the same time, the condom protects her from catching STI and HIV infections. Sheep membrane condoms are made from the intestines of lamb. The small pores in the condom do not let semen pass but they let certain bacteria and viruses through. Sheep membrane condoms therefore are only protective against pregnancy.

How effective is the condom in preventing unintended pregnancy?

Failure in this method is seldom due to the failure of the method itself, meaning failure due to the break of a condom.

All condoms on the Canadian market are tested for their quality. Condoms are very effective in preventing pregnancy when used consistently and correctly. Tests have shown that the percentage of women who become pregnant within the first year of perfect use of condoms is 3%. This means that out of 100 couples who used condoms correctly for 1 year, 3 couples experienced a pregnancy. The typical use failure rate is 12%. The typical use failure rate takes the misuse or non-use of the method into account. The highest failure rate is reported in women between ages 20-24.

Does the condom protect against sexually transmitted infections and HIV?

Latex condoms protect against STIs and HIV; sheep membrane condoms do not. A word of caution: Latex condoms may not fully protect against herpes and the human papillomaviruses (HPV) which causes genital warts. The reason is that these viruses are spread by skin to skin contact and are found in skin areas that are not covered by the condom. It is also a good idea to use a spermicide with a condom.

How popular are condoms in Canada?

In the 1998 Canadian Contraception Study, condoms were used by 22% of respondents.

Added value: Health benefits of the condom

Condoms offer a whole lot of benefits, which make them a great method. They can be used alone or in combination with another method and they have even more to offer than just protection against pregnancy, STIs and HIV.

Improving sexual relationships The condom can help men from ejaculating too fast. The use of the condom needs some practice and it can lead to better control of the time of ejaculation, which can help the woman to reach orgasm as well.

Protection against infertility Considering the danger of becoming infertile when infected with STIs, we can say that condoms protect against infertility by protecting against STIs.

Certain protection against cervical cancer Cervical cancer is associated with some viruses (HPV and herpes). The condom prevents the transmission of some of these viruses.

More hygienic The condom prevents semen from entering the vagina. The discharge after intercourse does not occur when using a condom.

Not convinced yet? Think of this.

Here are more features that make condoms a great method:

- Easy to get and relatively inexpensive.
- Great variety available to make the method more fun.
- Discreet to carry.
- Possible enhancement of erection.
- Prevents development of sperm allergy in women.
- Condom can be part of sex play and both partners can participate.
- Immediate, visible proof of effectiveness.

You are right, there are some flaws as well.
Condom use :

- Requires motivation, practice and sense of responsibility.
- May reduce sensitivity.
- May interfere with erection.
- May interrupt foreplay.
- May interfere with enjoyment.
- May cause embarrassment.
- May give unpleasant taste.

Where do I get condoms?
Nothing is easier than buying condoms. They are available in vending machines in washrooms, in drugstores, supermarkets, convenience stores, on-line and in condom shops.

What condoms are available in Canada?
They come in :

- Dry or lubricated form.
- With spermicide or without.
- Plain or reservoir-tipped.
- Straight or shaped.
- Smooth or textured.
- Different colours and different tastes.
- Different sizes (small, medium and large).

There are even condoms with an applicator on the market.

It can be so much fun
It's a matter of trying and checking out what you and your partner prefer. Condoms are by far the most fun method of contraception because the choice of models is so great. When you and your partner become familiar and comfortable with the use of condoms you have a wealth of possibilities to choose from. Different models might help you to improve your sex life! Get started and check it out!

A word of caution:
Always read the package insert! Some sophisticated models (special taste, special colour) have undergone certain treatments that make them less protective. This is clearly marked on the pack. The quality of latex can deteriorate with certain treatments, which are indicated in the inserts. The material also deteriorates when it comes into contact with oil-based products, such as Vaseline (petroleum jelly), and medicated vaginal creams.

1998 Canadian Contraception Study: CONTRACEPTION AND FIRST SEX

- Of all Canadian women aged 15-45 who had experienced sexual intercourse, 75% had used a method of contraception the first time they had intercourse.

- Approximately 70% of unmarried Canadian women under the age of 35 reported that they used a condom at first intercourse.

1. Check expiry date. When condoms are expired they do not protect any more.

2. Check the package. It should be sealed and not ripped. Do not use unpackaged condoms because the exposure to light weakens them.

3. Do not do any of your own testing like filling them with water or blowing a balloon to check whether they are intact! Experts have already done this! Your own testing might damage the condom!

4. Trial makes you the master. In the privacy of your bedroom, follow the instructions and apply the condom on the erect penis. Do this BEFORE you practice it with your partner. It will give you more self-assurance and will make it easier when it's time for the real thing! Try to put on the condom when it is dark or with your eyes closed as well.

5. Put a drop of water-based lubricant or saliva in the condom.

6. Place the rolled condom over the tip of the erect penis.

7. Leave a centimeter space at the tip of the condom to collect the semen if the condom does not already have a reservoir at the tip.

8. If not circumcised, pull back the foreskin with one hand.

9. Pinch the air out of the tip.

10. Unroll the condom over the penis. Unroll it all the way down to the base of the penis.

11. Smooth out any air bubbles.

12. Lubricate the outside of the penis before entering the vagina.

13. After ejaculation: be careful not to spill any semen. Hold the condom on the base of the penis while pulling out of the vagina. Pull out before the penis softens!

14. Throw the condom in the trash.

15. Wash penis with water and soap before any further contact.

16. Use a new condom each time you have intercourse!

TROUBLESHOOTING

The most common complaints with condoms are that they interfere with the sex play and that they decrease sensitivity. All of this need not happen if you and your partner are willing to put some effort into practicing! You should try different models until you find the right one that suits you!

Other problems might be...

My partner does not like to use a condom

This is a tough one...you have to convince your partner. Be creative! Here are some selling tools for you:
- One of you might have an STI without knowing or feeling anything at all.
- STIs and HIV infections can happen to anybody, no matter who you are.
- The majority of STIs are potentially more damaging to the woman than to the man. That's because many STIs infect the reproductive organs of the woman and may lead to infertility.

Losing the erection

A woman should always be supportive if the partner has a problem with his erection. After all, the man is showing responsibility by using a condom and the woman should encourage this. Putting on the condom could be part of making love. Masturbation and oral pleasuring techniques might help.

Condoms do not allow for spontaneity

If you and your partner make condom use a part of your sex play, there shouldn't be any problem with spontaneity.

Condom breaks

This very rarely happens with the condoms that are available today. Condom breakage also does not necessarily lead to pregnancy. Reasons for breakage are rough handling, use of an oil-based lubricant or expired condoms. Refer to the next page for advice and consult a physician or clinic for emergency contraception as soon as possible!

Condom slips off during intercourse

It can happen when too much lubricant was used on the inside of the condom. Take it off completely and use a new one with less lubricant. Consult a physician or clinic for emergency contraception as soon as possible!

IMPORTANT
- Use a condom **EVERY** time you have sex.
- Use a **NEW** condom for each act of intercourse.
- Keep the condoms in a dark and dry place away from heat.
- Always have a spermicide with an applicator handy to use with the condom and to use in an emergency when the condom slips or breaks. As the next step contact your physician or clinic for emergency contraception.
- Use only water-based lubricants with the condom. Please refer to the next page for different lubricants.
- For mouth to penis contact use condoms which are dry (not pre-treated with a lubricant) to avoid bad taste.

LUBRICANTS AND PRODUCTS THAT ARE SAFE OR UNSAFE TO USE WITH CONDOMS

SAFE

- Aloe-9
- Aqua-Lube & Aqua-Lube Plus
- Astroglide
- Carbowax
- Condom-mate
- Contraceptive foams (e.g. Delfen)
- Contraceptive creams and gels (e.g. Ramses)
- Duragel
- Egg white
- Foreplay lubricant
- Glycerin usp
- Intercept
- Koromex
- Lubafax
- Lubrin insert
- Ortho-Gynol
- Personal lubricant
- Prepair lubricant
- Probe
- Semicid
- Silicone DC 360
- Transi-Lube
- Saliva
- Water

UNSAFE

- Baby oils
- Burn ointments
- Coconut oil/butter
- All oils (peanut, sunflower, olive, corn…)
- Fish oils
- Hemorrhoid ointments
- Insect repellents
- Margarine, butter
- Mineral oil
- Palm oil
- Vaseline (petroleum jelly)
- Rubbing alcohol
- Suntan oil
- Vaginal creams (Monistat, Esterase, Femstat, Vagisil, Premarin, Rendell's Cone, Pharmatex Ovule)
- Some sexual lubricants (e.g. Elbow Grease, Hot Elbow Grease, Shaft)

RECOMMENDATIONS FOR CONDOM BREAKAGE AND SLIPPAGE

➡ Immediately insert spermicidal foam or gel.
➡ If no spermicide product is available, immediately wash both penis and vagina with soap and water.
➡ Emergency contraception.

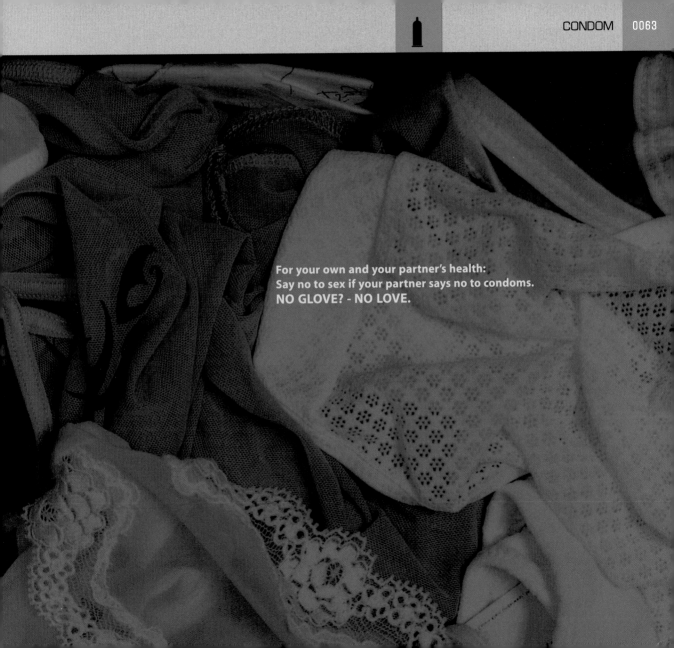

For your own and your partner's health:
Say no to sex if your partner says no to condoms.
NO GLOVE? - NO LOVE.

FEMALE CONDOM

IN A NUTSHELL

What is the female condom all about?
A polyurethane sheath with two rings for women to wear during vaginal intercourse. It protects against pregnancy, STIs and HIV.

What makes the female condom so special?
It is the only contraceptive controlled by women that protects against pregnancy and STI/HIV.

Does the female condom protect against sexually transmitted infections and HIV?
Yes

How effective is the female condom in preventing unintended pregnancy?
Used perfectly and consistently it has a failure rate of 5%.

How do I get it?
Prescription-free in drugstores, family planning clinics or on-line.

How do I use it?
Insert it in the vagina before intercourse. Insertion can be done hours before intercourse.

If you use a lubricant
Water or oil-based lubricants.

How much does it cost?
$12 for a pack of 3 condoms.

Possible problems
· Insertion difficulties.
· Sound during lovemaking.

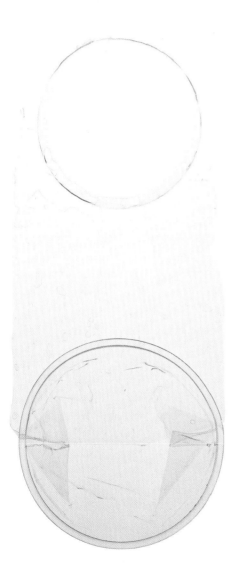

WHAT IS THE FEMALE CONDOM ALL ABOUT?

It is a polyurethane sheath, which is a thin and supple kind of plastic. When you compare it with condoms made for men:

- It does not contain latex.
- It is bigger in size because it has to fit the size of the vagina.
- It has two rings. The inner ring at the closed end of the condom is used to insert the condom and to keep it in place. It slides in place behind the pubic bone, acting like an anchor for the condom. The outer ring remains outside the vagina and partially covers and protects the lips of the vagina.

There is only one brand available in Canada, which is called Reality Female Condom. It is the only method controlled by the woman that provides double protection: it protects against unintended pregnancy and STIs.

How does it work?

The woman places the female condom into her vagina before intercourse, or more precisely, before any vaginal contact with the partner. The condom fits against the walls of the vagina and has a double effect:

- It prevents the semen from getting into the vagina.
- It prevents the exchange of body fluids between both partners.
- The outer ring of the condom protects the lips at the entrance of the vagina. The female condom offers good protection against unintended pregnancy and is a great barrier against sexually transmitted infections.

How effective is the female condom in preventing unintended pregnancy?

When used properly and consistently it is as effective as the male condom. Statistically speaking, only 5 out of 100 women using the female condom correctly over a period of one year may become pregnant.

(?)   **Can the condom disappear inside the vagina?**

The outer ring holds it in place even if movements become very intense during intercourse. The condom can be removed easily after intercourse by pulling with two fingers. However, if it disappears you have to interrupt lovemaking and put it back in place.

(?)   **Can I pass urine while the condom is in place?**

No problem. The urine passes through the urethra, a different canal than the vagina. It is above the vagina, under the pubic bone. You can interrupt lovemaking at any time to go to the washroom, leaving the condom in place.

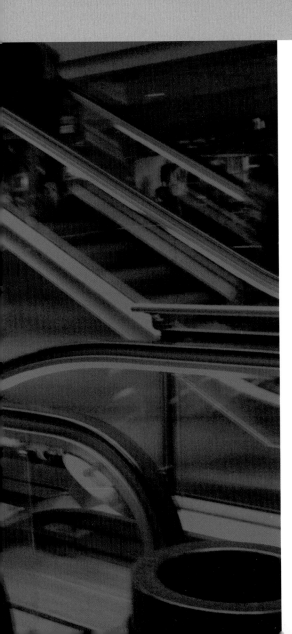

Does the female condom protect against sexually transmitted infections and HIV?

YES. This is the only contraceptive controlled by the female that protects against sexually transmitted infections and HIV.

How popular is the female condom in Canada?

In the 1998 Canadian Contraception Study, the female condom was used by 1% of respondents. This low rate is due to a lack of awareness about the many advantages of this method, which was only recently approved in Canada. Nearly all Canadian women in the age group 15-45 were aware of the pill and the condom, but only 25% were familiar with the female condom.

Where do I get the female condom?

In the drugstore or on-line. You do not need a prescription.

1999 Global Sex Survey:
HOW SOON DO YOU HAVE SEX AFTER GETTING TO KNOW YOUR PARTNER?

- 4% had sex on their first date
- 9% within the first week
- 38% within the first month
- 24% within the first 3 months
- 12% within the first 6 months
- 13% after 6 months
- 9% had sex only after getting married

1 Study the package insert. It sounds like a boring idea but the package insert contains illustrations and very good explanations.

2 Trial makes you the master. Use one condom and insert it as directed. In the heat of the moment when you are planning to have intercourse you do not want to go to the bathroom and read the instructions first.

3 Talk to your partner about trying it.

Let's talk about it!

It is a good idea to tell your partner about this method before you use it for the first time with him. This way you can prepare him, and you will not have any discussion in the middle of lovemaking! If your partner normally uses a condom you will have to tell him that he cannot use it when you use the female condom. Two condoms together do not work!

Here are some important things to remember:

➡ Use the female condom every time you have sex.

➡ Use a new condom with each sex act. After ejaculation you have to remove the condom BEFORE standing up and throw it in the garbage. (Not into the toilet because it might block it!)

➡ Guide the penis into the outer ring to make sure that it does not go on the side, passing the condom by.

➡ Good lubrication inside the condom is important for a smooth ride! Use more lubricant if the penis sticks to the condom and cannot move freely. You can even use lotion or other oil-based products if you do not have water-based lubricants with you.

SPECIAL FEATURES OF THE FEMALE CONDOM

The female condom was introduced in Canada in 1996. What is true for many things is especially true for the female condom: you won't know if you'll like it unless you really try it! Here are some features of the condom that might spark your interest:

· The female condom is an excellent alternative if your male partner does not like to use a condom because of a latex allergy or because of general dislike.

· People with a latex allergy can use the female condom because it is made out of polyurethane.

· The condom is made out of a very thin plastic, which warms up instantly to body temperature. It is thinner than the usual male condoms and allows for a more natural feeling and sensitivity during lovemaking.

· The condom has a lubricant on the outside and inside. The outside lubricant combines with the natural lubrication in the vagina and makes the condom fit against the walls of the vagina. The inside lubricant helps the penis to enter the condom.

- Unlike the condom worn by the male, the female condom is spacious and does not fit tightly on the penis. This is a great advantage considering that some men don't like to use a condom because they feel it is too tight on their penises.

- To make the entry of the penis into the vagina easier you can use water, or oil-based lubricants or moisturizers. There are sachets of extra lubricant that come with the female condom in the same pack.

- The condom can be inserted hours before intercourse, meaning you do not have to interrupt lovemaking. This is a great advantage considering that the condom used by the male partner can only be put on during sex when the penis is erect.

- After intercourse you can take your time before removing the condom. It does not have to be done immediately afterwards but before standing up.

TROUBLESHOOTING

The most common complaint with the female condom is difficulty with the insertion (that's why we highly recommend that you practice!). Others might be...

The condom makes noise

Obviously it cannot make noise on its own; it depends on the action! Relax! This can even be fun. The noise depends on the shape of the vagina, which is responsible for the fit of the condom. It also depends on the movement of the penis in the vagina. You can always try the following to change the noise: change the position during lovemaking. You may also want to add more lubricant on the inside.

The condom breaks

This is very unlikely because the material the female condom is made of is about 40% stronger than the latex condom. Because of this quality soon there will be another male condom on the market made out of the same material as the female condom.

If a condom breaks you might be in for some adventure. Use an applicator and apply spermicide into the vagina immediately. Refer to Chapter 8 on emergency contraception.

CONTRACEPTIVE SPONGE

What is the contraceptive sponge all about?
A disposable barrier made out of polyurethane foam, which is placed at the cervix. It absorbs and traps sperm. For additional protection against pregnancy the sponge contains a mix of three spermicides that destroy sperm.

What makes the sponge so special?
- It is a barrier method and a spermicide in one product.
- Very low concentration of spermicides make irritation in the vagina very unlikely.
- 12-hour protection against pregnancy.
- No change of sponge necessary if intercourse is repeated within the 12-hour period.

Does the sponge protect against sexually transmitted infections and HIV?
Yes, to a certain extent. For full protection the sponge has to be used in combination with a male condom. However, the spermicides in the sponge could provide protection against some STIs. Tests regarding a possible protection against HIV are ongoing.

How effective is the sponge in preventing unintended pregnancy?
Used perfectly the probability of failure during the first year of use is 11 %.

How do I get it?
Prescription-free in drugstores, family planning clinics, on-line.

How much does it cost?
Around $10 for a box of four Protectaid sponges.

Possible problems
- Difficulties in removing the sponge.
- Forgetting to take out the sponge.
- Allergy against the foam or the spermicides.

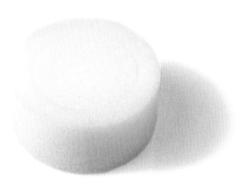

Actual size

WHAT IS THE CONTRACEPTIVE SPONGE ALL ABOUT?

It is a disposable, one-size-fits-all polyurethane foam device that fits over the cervix. The sponge is round and has two slots for the hand to fit in to make insertion and removal easy. There is only one product available in Canada, which is called Protectaid.

How does the contraceptive sponge work?
It is inserted into the vagina to cover the entrance of the uterus (cervix). The sponge does two things:

- It acts as a barrier to prevent the sperm from entering the cervix by absorbing and trapping sperm.
- The sponge contains F-5 Gel, a combination of spermicides that destroy sperm. The spermicides are nonoxynol-9, benzalkonium chloride and sodium cholate.

The concentrations of these three spermicides are very low, reducing the possibility of irritation in the vaginal wall and on the penis. The sponge provides protection for 12 hours.

How effective is the sponge in preventing unintended pregnancy?
There is a slight difference in efficacy between women who have already given birth (parous) and women who have not (nulliparous). A multinational study on Protectaid revealed that after one year of typical use, 21% of nulliparous women and 26% of parous women became pregnant. This difference was not statistically significant. The overall failure rate for perfect use was 11%.

Out of 100 women who used the sponge during a one-year period (and not always correctly), 21 women became pregnant in the group who had not given birth, and 26 became pregnant in the group that had.

When the sponge is used in combination with the male condom the efficacy rises dramatically to a failure rate of only 2%.

Does the sponge protect against sexually transmitted infections and HIV?
The sponge should be used in combination with a male latex condom. However, there is some evidence that the mix of three spermicides in the sponge can destroy certain bacteria and viruses including chlamydia and HIV. Research is ongoing and until new data becomes available a male condom should be used during sex. Practice safer sex: use double protection!

How popular is the sponge in Canada?
Protectaid was introduced in 1996. The other sponges (Today and Pharmatex) are not marketed in Canada any more. They contained higher concentrations of spermicides which led to skin irritations.

In the 1998 Canadian Contraception Study, the sponge was used by 1% of respondents.

Where do I get the sponge?
Prescription-free in the drugstore, in a family planning clinic or on-line.

(1) Check expiry date.

(2) Read the package insert.

(3) Wash hands with soap before touching sponge and inserting it.

(4) Practice the insertion for yourself.

(5) Keep timing in mind: insert at least 15 minutes before intercourse; take it out at the earliest 6 hours after intercourse.

(6) Do not use a vaginal douche with the sponge in place.

(7) Throw the used sponge in the trash.

(8) NEVER reuse a sponge.

Important points to keep in mind:

→ Use a sponge every time you have sex.

→ Never reuse a sponge.

→ Practice! Insertion needs some practice.

→ Do not use during menstruation.

→ Do not forget to take it out! It may be forgotten and left in place because it cannot be felt: potential risk for toxic shock syndrome.

SPECIAL FEATURES OF THE SPONGE

Here are some facts which make it an interesting alternative to other methods:

Timing:

- Sponge can be inserted hours before intercourse.
- Insert sponge at least 15 minutes before lovemaking.
- Sponge provides continuous protection for 12 hours.
- No new sponge needed if another act of intercourse happens within 12 hours.
- After intercourse: leave the sponge in place for a minimum of 6 hours.

Action:

- Sponge has a double action (spermicide to destroy sperm and barrier against sperm).
- No systemic reactions.
- Could provide some STI protection.

Convenience:

- Easy to carry.
- Prescription-free.
- No fitting, no physician required.
- Insertion does not interrupt sex play.
- Sponge cannot be felt by either partner.
- No leakage of semen through the vagina after ejaculation because the sponge absorbs semen.

TROUBLESHOOTING

The following problems might occur and they could be a signal to you to make an appointment with your physician.

Odour

If there is an unpleasant smell after removing the sponge, do not be concerned. Any material placed in the vagina that comes into contact with vaginal fluids and possibly semen will smell. However, if the sponge has a different colour than before and the smell from the vagina stays even for days after removal of the sponge, you should make an appointment with a physician.

Yeast infection/Bacterial vaginosis

Some sponge users have a problem with recurrent yeast infections and bacterial vaginosis. You should ask your physician whether you should consider another method of contraception. However, clinical studies with Protectaid did not show any increased incidence of infections with long-term use.

Allergy against spermicides or polyurethane

If you develop an allergic reaction to any of the ingredients that make up a sponge you will have to consider another method.

Toxic shock syndrome (TSS)

This is a very serious and very rare medical condition that you might have heard about in reference to tampon use during menstruation. Do not leave the sponge in the vagina for longer than 12 hours. If you experience two or more of the warning signs you have to go to the emergency room of a hospital immediately:

- Sudden high fever
- Diarrhoea
- Vomiting
- Dizziness
- Weakness
- Muscle aches
- Fainting or near fainting
- Sunburn-like rash in the palms of the hands or on the soles of the feet

LEA CONTRACEPTIVE

What is the Lea contraceptive all about?
A soft and pliable barrier device made out of silicone. The device is designed in such a way that it stays in place during intercourse. It should be used with a spermicide. It stops the sperm from entering the cervix.

What makes the Lea contraceptive so special?
- 8-hour protection against pregnancy.
- Very private, the contraceptive can be inserted hours before being with your partner.
- It has to be used with a spermicide.
- You can reuse it.

Does it protect against sexually transmitted infections and HIV?
No. The device itself is not protective. The spermicide added to it by the user protects against bacterial infections. The protection against viral infections, such as HIV has not been proven.

How effective is the Lea contraceptive in preventing unintended pregnancy?
Actual failure rates for typical use: 8.7% when used in combination with a spermicide, 12.9% when used alone.

How do I get it?
Prescription-free in drugstores, family planning clinics, or on-line.

How do I use it?
Insert it through the vagina and place it in front of the cervix before intercourse.

If you use a lubricant
Only water-based lubricants.

How much does it cost?
Approximately $50.

Possible problems
- Allergy against silicone or against the spermicide you use in combination with it.
- Insertion difficulties.

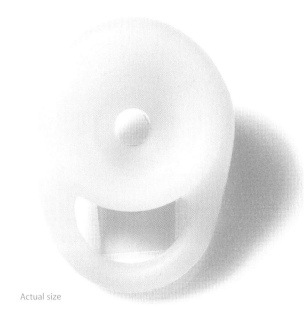

Actual size

WHAT IS THE LEA CONTRACEPTIVE ALL ABOUT?

It is a soft, pliable barrier contraceptive made of silicone. It is a cup-shaped bowl with a valve and a loop. The loop is for easy insertion and removal. The shape of this barrier device is designed to keep the barrier in place. The Lea contraceptive should be used in combination with a spermicide.

How does the Lea contraceptive work?
It is inserted through the vagina to the front of the cervix to surround the cervix without resting on it. The contraceptive acts as a barrier to prevent the sperm from entering the cervix. It is used with a spermicide, which destroys the sperm on contact. The device is one-size only.

How effective is the Lea contraceptive in preventing unintended pregnancy?
The failure rate for typical use is 8.7% when used with a spermicide. Typical use implies that some people in the study did not use the device correctly. When used without a spermicide (not recommended!) the failure rate is higher: 12.9%.

Does it protect against sexually transmitted infections and HIV?
No. The male latex condom should be used in addition to the Lea contraceptive to protect both partners from STIs and HIV. Practice safer sex: use double protection!

Where do I get the Lea contraceptive?
Prescription-free in the drugstore, on-line or in a family planning clinic. More than likely you will not find it on the shelf. Ask the pharmacist and he/she will be able to order it for you.

Storage and care
After taking it out, wash it with water and soap, dry it with a towel and store it in the plastic pouch that comes with the product. Use a cotton swab to clean the area with the valve. The silicone can start to yellow after 6 months.

① Read the package insert.

② Practice the insertion for yourself.

③ Wear it for a while and get comfortable with it. You should not feel the device inside you.

④ Remove it. Insert your index finger and grasp the loop. Once the finger is holding the loop, twist until suction is broken. Pull it down and out of the vagina.

Avoid common mistakes and do the following:

➡ Wash hands with soap before taking the Lea contraceptive out of the plastic bag and inserting it.

➡ Coat the inside of the bowl (one-third full) with spermicidal gel. If you use too much spermicide the insertion will be very difficult because it becomes too slippery.

➡ Also apply a small amount of gel around the thickest part of the bowl to make insertion easier.

➡ Insert the Lea contraceptive as directed in the package insert before intercourse.

➡ After intercourse: leave the Lea contraceptive in place for a minimum of 8 hours.

➡ The contraceptive should not stay in the vagina longer than 24 hours.

SPECIAL FEATURES OF THE LEA CONTRACEPTIVE

Here are some facts which make it an interesting alternative to other methods:

Timing:

- Can be inserted hours before intercourse.
- Should be left in place at least 8 hours after the last act of intercourse.
- Should not be worn longer than 24 hours in a row.

Convenience:

- Continuous protection for 8 hours.
- It can be reused over a period of 6 months when taken care of properly.
- No special skills and preparations required.
- Easy to carry, easy to get.
- No fitting, no physician required.
- Insertion does not interrupt sex play.
- No systemic reactions.
- Can be used during menstruation.

TROUBLESHOOTING

CAUTION

- The woman must be comfortable with touching her vagina to insert the Lea contraceptive.

- Insertion and removal needs some practice at first.

The contraceptive can be felt by the partner during intercourse

This can happen when it is not inserted correctly. Read the instructions again and try another time! The Lea contraceptive should not be felt by either partner.

Foul odour

If you notice a foul odour while the device is in place or after removing it, contact your physician. It could be an infection.

Toxic shock syndrome (TSS) ⚠

Do not leave the Lea contraceptive in the vagina for longer than 24 hours. For TSS danger signs go to page 73.

DIAPHRAGM

What is the diaphragm all about?
A flat latex cap with an enclosed ring, which fits against the cervix. It prevents sperm from entering the uterus. The diaphragm has to be used in combination with a spermicide (gel or cream). The spermicide destroys the sperm.

What makes the diaphragm so special?
- A very private method because the diaphragm can be inserted before intercourse.
- The insertion needs some practice and a motivated user.
- Has to be used with a spermicide and you can reuse it.

Does it protect against sexually transmitted infections and HIV?
No. The diaphragm itself is not protective. The spermicide added to it by the user protects against bacterial infections. The protection against viral infections, such as HIV has not been proven.

How effective is the diaphragm in preventing unintended pregnancy?
Used perfectly the probability of failure during the first year of use is 4 - 8%.

If you want to use a lubricant
Only water-based products.

What makes it different from the cervical cap?
- It is bigger.
- It is easier to insert.
- It needs more spermicide.
- Higher risk of urinary tract infections.
- Can be used during menstruation.

How do I get it?
You need an appointment with your family physician, gynaecologist or family planning clinic to get a diaphragm fitted for your body.

How do I use it?
Insert the diaphragm by hand through the vagina in front of the cervix anytime before intercourse.

How much does it cost?
Around $40.

Possible problems
Sensitivity or allergies towards latex or spermicides are reasons not to use it. Women suffering from urinary tract infections (UTI) should not use it. There is a possibility of developing a UTI while using the diaphragm. Insertion problems. Wrong fit.

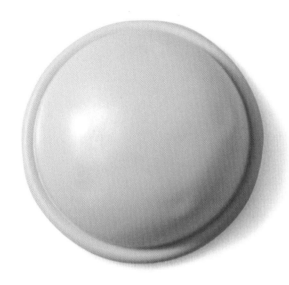

Actual size

WHAT IS THE DIAPHRAGM ALL ABOUT?

A diaphragm is a latex cap that covers the cervix. It has a flexible steel ring on the edge to help keep its shape. The steel ring is surrounded by rubber and cannot cause any harm. This barrier method has to be used in combination with a spermicide (gel or cream) to give sufficient protection against pregnancy.

How does the diaphragm work?

The woman has to place the diaphragm through the vagina to the front of the cervix. There the diaphragm acts like a barrier and prevents sperm from going through. During intercourse the vagina is moving and the diaphragm is not always a perfect seal on the cervix. This is why the diaphragm has to be used with a spermicide to increase protection against pregnancy.

How effective is the diaphragm in preventing unintended pregnancy?

If used perfectly (meaning it fits you well and you use it every time you have sex) the failure rate during the first year of use is 4-8 %. In other words: of 100 women who used the diaphragm consistently and correctly during one year, 4-8 became pregnant.

Does the diaphragm protect against sexually transmitted infections and HIV?

It does not fully protect because there is still an exchange of body fluids (semen and natural lubrication of the vagina) between partners. However, there is a reduced risk of bacterial infection due to the fact that semen does not enter the cervix. The spermicide protects against STIs caused by bacteria, however, protection against viral infections such as HIV has not been proven. The male partner should use a latex condom to protect both partners from a possible infection. Practice safer sex: use double protection!

How popular is the diaphragm in Canada?

In the 1998 Canadian Contraception Study, the diaphragm was used by 1% of respondents.

Where do I get a diaphragm?

You have to make an appointment with your family physician, gynaecologist or family planning clinic. A pelvic exam and a medical history will be taken. For more information refer to page 28. The pelvic exam is necessary to fit you with the right type and size of diaphragm. The size and type will depend upon your build and whether or not you have had children. The physician will explain how to insert it and will let you insert it yourself in the changing room. Afterwards he/she will check whether it fits well and if you have inserted it correctly. The sure sign that it fits well is that you do not feel it at all. With the prescription you can buy the diaphragm at the pharmacy and use it for years when you take care of it properly.

What types of diaphragms are available in Canada?

There are two different types available in Canada and they are offered in various sizes.

Storage and care

Wash it with warm water and mild soap, dry it and put it back in the box. Keep it away from light and excessive heat. Keep the storage box in a place where you will find it afterwards (with your toothbrush for example). The empty box will remind you to take the diaphragm out and will save you from forgetting! Replace it when it is damaged or bent. It is good for a year or two if you look after it well!

**1999 Global Sex Survey:
BARRIER METHODS FOR THE
ADVENTUROUS**

34% of sexually active young adults (40% of the men, 28% of the women), said they had experienced a sexual relationship with more than one partner at a time.

SPECIAL FEATURES OF THE DIAPHRAGM

Here are some facts that make it an interesting alternative to other methods:

Timing:

You can insert the diaphragm anytime before intercourse. This is an advantage because you do not have to bother about it when you are in the middle of lovemaking. It has to be left inside the vagina for a minimum of 8 hours after intercourse. It should not be worn longer than 24 hours.

Action:

You have to use a spermicide with the diaphragm. For each repeated act of intercourse you will have to use additional spermicide using an applicator while leaving the device in place.

Caution:

If you or your partner have a problem with latex products you should not use this method.

Be motivated:

You have to carry your diaphragm with you and you always have to have spermicidal gel or cream with an applicator handy!

1 Study the package insert. It sounds like a boring idea but the package insert contains helpful illustrations and very good explanations.

2 Trial makes you the master. Insert it as directed. In the heat of the moment when you are planning to have intercourse you do not want to go to the bathroom, read the instructions and get all nervous.

3 Walk around with the diaphragm in place. Do some exercises and make sure you do not feel it. If you do feel it even when it is placed correctly you will have to contact your physician and get it exchanged.

4 Take it out, wash it and try it again. For the removal: Insert a finger in the vagina, locate the rim of the diaphragm. Hook the finger behind it and pull it out.

5 Better be safe than sorry. The first few times you use the diaphragm your partner should use a condom until you are sure you get it right!

Avoid common mistakes and do the following:

➡ Use the diaphragm EVERY time you have sex, also during your period.

➡ Wash your hands before touching and inserting the diaphragm.

➡ Hold it against the light to check for holes and tears. If there is any damage it does not protect you.

➡ Check expiry date of spermicide.

➡ Apply a spermicide before insertion.

➡ Insert the diaphragm (you know how, practiced before, right?).

➡ Apply more spermicide after each act of intercourse without taking the diaphragm out. You need a spermicide with an applicator to reach into the vagina for that.

➡ If you want to use a lubricant or moisturizer, use only water-based lubricants or moisturizers.

➡ Wait 8 hours after intercourse to take it out. You do not have to set an alarm clock for this but the diaphragm should not stay in your vagina longer than 24 hours.

➡ Do not use a vaginal douche.

TROUBLESHOOTING

Difficulty with insertion

The most common complaint with the diaphragm is difficulty with the insertion (that's why we highly recommend that you practice!). One major mistake: too much spermicide! If the spermicide is all over the diaphragm it will become too slippery to handle when you fold it for insertion. The solution is: use only 1-2 teaspoons of spermicide (depends on size of the diaphragm) and PRACTICE!

Refitting necessary when...

You might need another size of diaphragm after giving birth, after an abortion or after surgery in the pelvis. You have to make an appointment with your physician.

Diaphragm goes out of place during lovemaking

In this case sperm from the pre-ejaculate or the ejaculate may have passed the barrier. Apply some more spermicide immediately. Contact your physician for emergency contraception.

Urinary tract infections (UTI)

Diaphragms can increase the risk of urinary tract infections due to the pressure of the flexible steel ring on the urethra. If you suffer from UTI (infections in the bladder or urethra that make it painful to pass urine) you better not use the diaphragm as a method of contraception. If you develop a UTI while using the diaphragm, your physician might prescribe another type for you (with another rim that puts less pressure on the urethra.)

Toxic shock syndrome (TSS)

Do not leave the diaphragm in the vagina for longer than 24 hours. For TSS danger signs go to page 73.

CERVICAL CAP

What is the cervical cap all about?
A deep latex cap that fits against the cervix. It prevents sperm and bacteria from entering the cervix. The cervical cap has to be used with spermicidal cream or gel. The spermicide destroys sperm.

What makes the cervical cap so special?
- A very private method, does not interfere with sex because it can be inserted before.
- Insertion needs some practice and requires a motivated user.
- Has to be used with a spermicide and you can reuse it.

Does it protect against sexually transmitted Infections and HIV?
No. The cervical cap itself is not protective. The spermicide added to it by the user protects against bacterial infections. The protection against viral infections, such as HIV, has not been proven.

How effective is the cervical cap in preventing unintended pregnancy?
Used perfectly, the probability of failure during the first year of use is 10-13%. A higher failure was reported in women who had already had a baby.

If you use a lubricant
Only water-based products.

What makes it different from the diaphragm?
- It is smaller.
- Insertion might need more practice.
- Requires less spermicide.
- Lower risk of urinary tract infections.
- Must not be used during menstruation.

How do I get it?
You need an appointment at a clinic or with your gynaecologist who will examine you to find out the correct size of cervical cap to fit you perfectly. You will get a prescription to buy the cap at a pharmacy or clinic.

How do I use it?
Insert it through the vagina in front of the cervix anytime before intercourse.

How much does it cost?
Around $40.

Possible problems
- A sensitivity or allergy towards rubber or spermicide is a reason not to use it. The annual Pap smear is important to check for possible inflammation in the cervix.
- Insertion problems.
- Wrong fit.

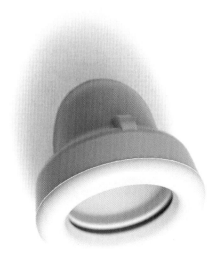

Actual size

WHAT IS THE CERVICAL CAP ALL ABOUT?

A cervical cap is a small latex cap with a flexible ring around the edge. It fits over the entrance of the cervix to prevent sperm from entering the uterus. This barrier method has to be used in combination with a spermicide applied before insertion of the cap (gel or cream) to give sufficient protection against unintended pregnancy.

How does the cervical cap work?

The woman has to push the cervical cap through the vagina and place it over the cervix. There the cervical cap acts like a barrier and prevents semen from entering. It is smaller than a diaphragm and it is held in place by suction. During intercourse the vagina is moving and the cap is not always a perfect seal on the cervix. For better protection the cervical cap has to be used with spermicidal cream or gel in and around the cap.

How effective is the cap in preventing unintended pregnancy?

There is a difference in effectiveness when used by women who have already given birth (parous) and women who have not (nulliparous). If used perfectly (meaning it fits you well and you insert the cap correctly every time you have sex) the failure rate during the first year of use is 10-13%. This means that over a one-year study, 10-13 pregnancies occurred in 100 couples who used the cervical cap. Studies have shown a higher failure rate in the first year of use among parous women (26-27%). The use of spermicidal cream or gel is very important to insure good protection against pregnancy.

The effectiveness of the cervical cap depends on the correct fit over the cervix and on the correct insertion by the woman. That's where your skills come in! Any event that might change the shape of the cervix (birth, abortion, and other surgery) makes a refitting of the cervical cap necessary.

Does the cap protect against sexually transmitted infections and HIV?

The cervical cap protects the fallopian tubes and the uterus from sperm and bacteria. The vagina and the penis are still exposed to body fluids such as sperm and the natural lubrication of the vagina.

To summarize:

- There is a reduced risk of bacterial infection due to the fact that sperm does not enter the cervix and because of the protective effect of the spermicide.
- Protection against viral infections such as HIV has not been proven. The male partner should use a condom to protect both partners from a possible infection.

Practice safer sex: use double protection!

How popular is the cervical cap in Canada?

In the 1998 Canadian Contraception Study, the cervical cap was used by 1% of respondents.

Where do I get a cervical cap?

You have to make an appointment with your family physician, gynaecologist or family planning clinic. Avoid the following time periods during which the fitting of the cap cannot be done:

- Within 6 weeks after giving birth.
- Within 6 weeks of an abortion or other pelvic surgery.
- During menstruation.

A pelvic exam and a medical history will be taken. For more information about the pelvic exam refer to page 28. A Pap smear will be performed to rule out any infections. The size and type of cervical cap will depend upon your build and whether or not you have had children. The cap has to fit the entrance of your cervix. After insertion it is kept in place by suction and for best protection it is important that it fits well. The physician will explain to you how to insert it and will let you insert it yourself in the changing room. Afterwards he/she will check whether it fits well and if you've inserted it correctly. The sure sign that it fits well is that you don't feel it at all. With the prescription you can buy the cervical cap at the pharmacy and use it for at least a year. A follow-up visit after 3 months is a good idea to check whether the method fits your lifestyle and to solve any problems you might have with it.

Storage and care

Wash it with warm water and mild soap, dry it with a cloth and put it back in the box. Keep it away from light and excessive heat. Keep the storage box in a place where you will find it afterwards (with your toothbrush for example). The empty box will remind you to take the cervical cap out and will save you from forgetting! Replace it when it is damaged or bent. With proper care it can last for years.

What types of cervical caps are available in Canada?

There is one type available, which comes in different sizes: Prentif Cap.

CAUTION!
THE CERVICAL CAP IS NOT FOR YOU IF:

- **You or your partner are allergic to spermicide or rubber.**
- **You just gave birth, had an abortion or other pelvic surgery.**

SPECIAL FEATURES OF THE CERVICAL CAP

Here are some facts, which make it an interesting alternative to other methods:

Timing:

You can insert the cap hours before intercourse. This is an advantage because you do not have to bother about it when you are in the middle of "things"...

Action:

Spermicidal gel or cream is a must. You have to use a spermicide with the cap at the time of insertion. For each repeated act of intercourse you should use additional spermicide while leaving the device in place. You need to have spermicidal cream or gel in an applicator to insert it into the vagina.

Be motivated:

You have to carry your cervical cap with you and you always have to have spermicidal cream or gel handy!

1 Study the package insert. It sounds like a boring idea but the package insert contains illustrations and very good explanations.

2 Trial makes you the master. Insert it as directed. In the heat of the moment when you are planning to have intercourse you do not want to go to the bathroom, read the instructions and get all nervous.

3 Walk around with the cervical cap in place. Do some exercises and make sure you do not feel it. If you feel it you will have to try again or see your physician to fit you with another size of cap.

4 Take it out, wash it and try it again. For removal: Insert a finger in the vagina, locate the cap rim, press on the rim until the seal against the cervix breaks and tilt it so it comes off the cervix. With the finger behind the rim, pull it out.

5 Better to be safe than sorry. Until you are really familiar and comfortable with the insertion of the cap, your partner should use a condom.

Avoid common mistakes and do the following:

→ Use the cervical cap EVERY time you have sex. If it sits in your drawer it cannot do its job!

→ Use another method during menstruation. Do not use the cap during menstruation.

→ Wash hands before touching and inserting the cap.

→ Hold it against the light to check for holes and tears. If there is any damage it will not protect you.

→ Check expiry date of spermicide.

→ Apply spermicidal cream or gel before insertion; don't fill more than 1/3 of the cap.

→ If necessary: use only water-based lubricants or moisturizers.

→ Insert it before intercourse so that a good seal around the cervix can develop.

→ Wait 8 hours after intercourse to take it out. You do not have to set an alarm clock for this but it should not be in your vagina longer than 24 hours.

→ Vaginal douche: not before 6 hours after the last act of intercourse.

TROUBLESHOOTING

Insertion problems

The most common complaint is difficulty with the insertion. That's why we highly recommend that you practice! One major mistake is the use of too much spermicide! If you fill more than 1/3 of the cap it will become too slippery to handle.

Foul smell and discharge

This might occur when you leave the cervical cap in place too long. Get into the habit of putting the storage box close to your toothbrush so you will remember when you brush your teeth that you still have the cap in your body. Leave it in place at least 8 hours after the last act of intercourse, but in total it shouldn't be left in place longer than 24 hours.

A trick: You can leave the cap in a water/chlorophyll solution for a few hours to get rid of a bad smell.

Cervical cap goes out of place during lovemaking

In this case sperm from the pre-ejaculate or the ejaculate may have passed the barrier. Apply more spermicide with an applicator immediately. Contact your physician for emergency contraception.

Toxic shock syndrome (TSS)

Do not leave the cervical cap in the vagina for longer than 24 hours. For TSS danger signs go to page 73.

SPERMICIDES

What are spermicides all about?
A chemical called nonoxynol-9, which comes in the form of cream, gel, foam, film or suppository. After insertion into the vagina in front of the cervix, it destroys sperm on contact. Spermicides should be used in combination with other methods, such as the condom. Some condoms already have a spermicide on them.

What make spermicides so special?
- There are many different brands available.
- It is a very effective method of contraception when used in combination with a barrier method such as diaphragm, cervical cap and condom.
- It offers protection against bacterial infections and pelvic inflammatory disease.
- It can be used as an emergency method after an "accident" with the condom, the diaphragm or the cap.
- It lubricates the vagina and makes penetration easier.

Do spermicides protect against sexually transmitted infections and HIV?
Yes, they offer some protection. They protect against bacterial infections. The protection against viral infections, such as HIV is yet to be determined. Research is ongoing.

How effective are spermicides in preventing unintended pregnancy?
79-94% effective when used alone. It becomes a very safe method when used with another barrier method.

How do I get it?
In the drugstore or on-line.

How do I use them?
Apply deep into the vagina before intercourse. When to apply before intercourse depends on the products.

How much does it cost?
Example: Advantage 24 (pack of 3) around $10. Delfen (20-25 applications) around $18.

Possible problems
Irritation of entrance of vagina or tip of penis is possible. Timing of the application; sometimes messy.

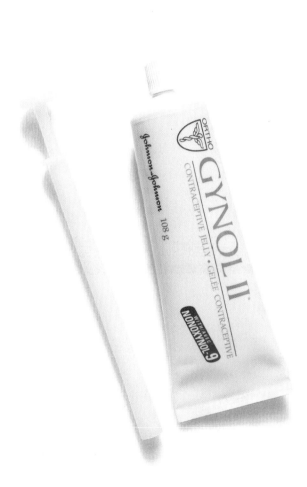

WHAT ARE SPERMICIDES ALL ABOUT?

Spermicides are chemicals that destroy sperm in the form of cream, gel, film, foam or suppository. The chemical agent used for spermicides is called nonoxynol-9. They can be used alone or together with the female condom, male condom, diaphragm, cervical cap and Lea contraceptive to increase protection against pregnancy. In an emergency situation (e.g. condom slips) spermicides can also be useful.

How do spermicides work?

Just before intercourse the woman applies spermicide in her vagina. The creams, gels or foams come with an applicator that helps to insert the substance deep into the vagina in front of the cervix. The male partner can also put spermicide directly on the condom. In fact, some condom brands already have spermicide on them. When sperm meets spermicide a chemical reaction takes place that destroys the sperm.

How effective are spermicides in preventing unintended pregnancy?

The consistent use of spermicides is the most important factor in minimizing failure! The failure rates of spermicides used alone range from 6% (perfect use) to 21% (typical use). The failure rate is lower when used by women who have a reduced fertility (e.g. over age 45). It is a very efficient method of contraception when it is used in combination with either a cervical cap, a diaphragm, Lea contraceptive, male or female condom. If spermicides are used with another barrier method, the protection against pregnancy is comparable to hormonal methods.

Here are some figures from a study performed in 1991. When condoms were used alone, the failure rate within the first year of use was 3%. When spermicides were used alone, the failure rate was 6%. When spermicide (applied separately) and condom were used together, the failure rate dropped to 0.01%.

SPERMICIDES: TYPES AND TIMING

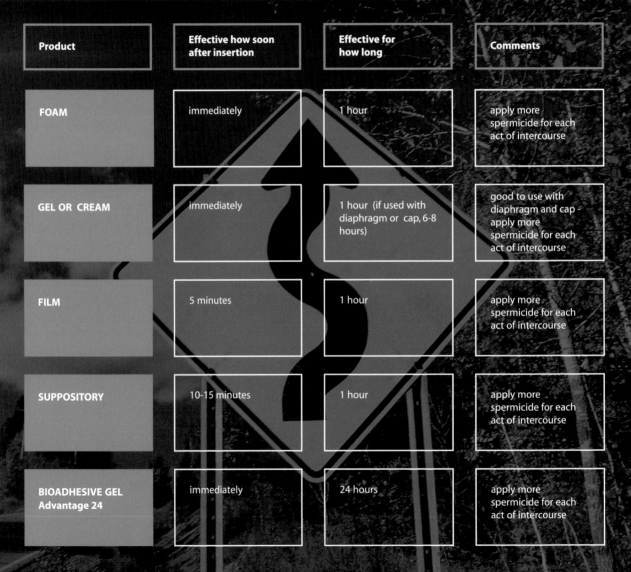

Product	Effective how soon after insertion	Effective for how long	Comments
FOAM	immediately	1 hour	apply more spermicide for each act of intercourse
GEL OR CREAM	immediately	1 hour (if used with diaphragm or cap, 6-8 hours)	good to use with diaphragm and cap - apply more spermicide for each act of intercourse
FILM	5 minutes	1 hour	apply more spermicide for each act of intercourse
SUPPOSITORY	10-15 minutes	1 hour	apply more spermicide for each act of intercourse
BIOADHESIVE GEL **Advantage 24**	immediately	24 hours	apply more spermicide for each act of intercourse

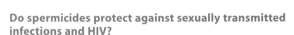

Do spermicides protect against sexually transmitted infections and HIV?

Spermicides protect against STIs caused by bacterial infections such as chlamydia and gonorrhoea. This is the main reason why spermicides have become very popular again in the past few years. Studies are ongoing to find out about the possible protection against viral infections such as HIV. Until further data becomes available, spermicides should only be used in combination with condoms in order to protect against STIs and HIV.

> # PRACTICE SAFER SEX:
> # USE DOUBLE PROTECTION!

How popular are spermicides in Canada?

In the 1998 Canadian Contraception Study, spermicides were used by 3% of respondents.

Added value: health benefits of spermicides

Spermicides offer certain benefits apart from contraception, which should spark your interest in trying:

- Spermicides reduce the risk for:
    - Pelvic inflammatory disease (PID) in women. PID can lead to infertility.
    - Bacterial infections such as chlamydia and gonorrhoea.
    - Cervical cancer, as some evidence suggests.
- Spermicides also offer a lubrication of the vagina which makes intercourse smoother (if the woman lacks lubrication in the vaginal walls). If the partner uses a condom it is also less likely to break because of the lubrication.
- Spermicides can be used in the following emergency situations to reduce the risk of becoming pregnant:
    - Dislocation of cervical cap or diaphragm during intercourse.
    - Breakage or leakage of condom.
- Spermicides have another big advantage. The woman can use them without the co-operation of her male partner. Unfortunately many women have difficulties convincing their partners to use condoms. With the use of spermicides the woman can have at least some protection against STIs.

Where do I get spermicides?

Prescription-free in drugstores, or for more privacy, on-line.

What spermicides are available in Canada?

Many different kinds and brands. Please refer to the table on the left to get an idea of the different types of spermicides.

The differences between cream, jelly, foam, suppository and film

There are a variety of products available. The differences between the products are important to know in order to make the right choice. You have to keep two things in mind:

1. Timing: when to apply the spermicide.
2. What other barrier method is being used.

Some products are effective immediately when you apply them, others need some time to become effective. This can interfere with you and your partner's way of lovemaking. The table on the left gives you a summary of the various types of products.

You also have to read the package insert of the other barrier method you are using in combination with the spermicide. If you use a diaphragm or a cervical cap, for example, you have to buy cream or gel. For the diaphragm you need a spermicide that comes with an applicator. The film and the foam work as well but they are not recommended with these methods. Condoms can be used with all spermicides.

1 Study the package insert. It sounds like a boring idea but the package insert contains good explanations. In this book we are only addressing the facts that apply to all spermicides on the market. But depending on which one you choose, you have to study the package insert for special instructions.

2 Trial makes you the master. For women: Insert it as directed. For men: Put some on top of your penis. This is to find out whether you are showing any allergic reactions.

3 Wait for the reaction. If you feel any irritation at the entrance of the vagina or on top of the penis, you might be allergic to the chemical and you will have to consider another method. But do not be too impatient. The feeling of irritation might disappear shortly and you are on your way!

Common mistakes and how to avoid them:
Correct placement and correct timing are important!

➡ Use spermicide EVERY time you have sex.

➡ Insert it high into the vagina following package instructions.

➡ Use the required amount (no less, no more, otherwise it becomes messy).

➡ Wait the time indicated until it becomes effective before starting lovemaking.

➡ Apply a new dose for every new act of intercourse.

➡ Do not use a vaginal douche afterwards (wait at least 6 hours).

➡ Always have a supply handy! For foam, cream and gel you also need an applicator. When you use foam, always have an extra container handy because you might not realize when a container is running low.

➡ If applicator is used: wash it with water and soap and store it after use.

A WORD ABOUT CONDOMS AND SPERMICIDES

Studies have shown that the protection against pregnancy is better when condoms are used together with an extra spermicide. Some condoms are pre-treated by the manufacturer, they have a spermicide on them already, but this is less effective.

WHAT ELSE IS NEW?

The newest product on the market, Advantage 24, has some special features that make it an innovative spermicide that is easy to handle:

- Disposable applicator with the right dose: You have the right dose ready and you do not have to reuse the applicator.
- It gives 24-hour protection: you can apply the spermicide long before lovemaking, which gives you more privacy (for the very active among you: for each repeated act of intercourse you have to apply a new dose!).
- Lower concentration of nonoxynol-9 leads to fewer irritations as compared to other spermicides.
- It has a built-in lubricant.

TROUBLESHOOTING

The most common complaint with spermicides is a burning sensation or an irritation on the woman's vulva or the man's penis. Other problems might be...

Problem with the timing

If you dislike waiting until the spermicide is effective, use foam, gel or cream because they are effective immediately after insertion. Have a look at the table on page 92 for a comparison. The new bioadhesive gel, Advantage 24, can even be inserted over 20 hours before intercourse.

Allergy

If you feel an allergic reaction when applying the spermicide you might be allergic to nonoxynol-9 (the spermicidal agent) or some other ingredient which is in the product. Try another product with different ingredients. They are marked on the package.

Unpleasant odour or taste

Just try different brands to find the one you and your partner like!

Messy

Suppositories, film and Advantage 24 are less messy. Use those.

This chapter is about the following methods:

Tubal Ligation

Vasectomy

SURGICAL METHODS
NO MORE KIDS- THAT'S IT!

Surgical methods are used by individuals who are seeking a permanent method of contraception. Reversal is in some cases impossible, and usually complicated and costly. Before choosing any of the two methods, tubal ligation or vasectomy, it is important that both partners in a couple discuss this step to prevent regret. We will provide you with all the necessary information to help you decide.

In the 1998 Canadian Contraception Study, surgical sterilization (male and female combined) was the second most frequently used method of contraception following the oral contraceptive pill.

TUBAL LIGATION DISCONNECTION THE FEMALE WAY

What is tubal ligation all about?
The two fallopian tubes, which transport the egg(s) after ovulation to the uterus, get disconnected. This way, after ovulation the egg cannot meet sperm and fertilization becomes impossible. A tubal ligation is considered permanent because a reversal is difficult, costly and not always successful.

What makes the method so special?
· It is the most effective method of contraception controlled by the woman apart from abstinence.
· It is for women who have completed their families and who do not want any other form of contraception (e.g. IUD).

Does it protect against sexually transmitted infections and HIV?
No

How effective is tubal ligation in preventing unintended pregnancy?
Pregnancy rates following tubal ligation are reported over a time period of 10 years following the surgery. They vary between 1 and 2.5% depending on the procedure chosen by the physician.

How do I get it?
You have to discuss it with your partner who should fully support your decision to have a tubal ligation. Then you have to see a gynaecologist who performs surgery. You can expect a full gynaecological exam and questions to make sure that you will not regret your decision. You will have to sign a consent form. When discussing this with your partner, keep in mind: A vasectomy, the male sterilization, is a much easier procedure and it involves fewer health risks.

How much does it cost?
It is usually covered by provincial health insurance plans.

Possible problems
Pain, bleeding, nausea following surgery. The biggest problem is regret. You have to keep in mind that this surgery makes a woman permanently sterile. The reversal is sometimes possible but does not always work out. Discuss it with your partner!

WHAT IS TUBAL LIGATION ALL ABOUT?

It is a surgical procedure that provides permanent contraception. It interrupts the journey of the female egg to the uterus. Tubal ligation (ligation=binding) is also referred to as female sterilization. To be sterile means to be unable to reproduce. It is considered to be a permanent method of contraception chosen mostly by women who have completed their families because the surgery is very difficult to reverse.

How does tubal ligation work?
During ovulation a ripe egg leaves one of the two ovaries, travels through the fallopian tube in direction of the uterus, and awaits the encounter of sperm in order to get fertilized. Tubal ligation disconnects both fallopian tubes and interrupts the transportation of the egg to the uterus. The procedure does not affect the daily work of the ovaries. The female cycle with its hormone production, ovulation and menstrual periods remains the same afterwards.

How effective is tubal ligation in preventing unintended pregnancy?
Pregnancy rates following tubal ligation are reported over a time period of 10 years following the surgery. They vary between 1 and 2.5% depending on the kind of procedure chosen by the physician. Studies have shown that the probability of failure for women sterilized at age 28 or younger is higher than in women who have the surgery past the age of 34.

Does tubal ligation protect against sexually transmitted infections and HIV?
No. Remember that there is no such thing as a free ticket to a worry-free love and sex life! It is handy to choose a method like sterilization, which effectively protects against pregnancy, but remember that it doesn't protect you from infections. If you and/or your partner are not mutually faithful to each other, or if you are at risk for STIs and HIV, you should use a male or female condom with a spermicide for protection.

Tubal ligation is a good choice for you, if:
- you and your partner are sure that you do not want to have more children or any children at all.
- you want a very effective, long-term method.
- you want a very private method.
- you want a method which is not related to intercourse.
- other (reversible) methods such as hormonal methods or the IUD are not options for you.

Tubal ligation is not for you, if:
- you are not sure that you want permanent contraception.
- your partner agrees to have a vasectomy because it is an easier procedure with fewer complications.

The 1998 Canadian Contraception Study revealed that:	
10%	of women in the study used the method
53%	of users were in the age group 30-44
40-44	is the age group in which tubal ligation is most popular

PRACTICE SAFER SEX: USE DOUBLE PROTECTION!

1 First of all, if you have a partner you should discuss this choice with him.

2 Ask your family physician, gynaecologist or family planning clinic where you should go for the tubal ligation.

3 Only gynaecologists who perform surgery do tubal ligations.

> To avoid later regret, it is important to have the support and consent of your partner for this method of contraception more than for any other.

What to expect when getting a tubal ligation?

Firstly, the physician who will perform the procedure will ask you questions. Please read the following paragraph to be prepared for some of the questions. It is very important to be absolutely sure that you want a tubal ligation because it is, in principle, a method of no return! You will have to sign a consent form.

Second, you will be examined to check whether this procedure can be done for you. The physician will want to find out whether he or she can easily access the tubes, whether you have any infections, or whether you are pregnant. You will also get information about the possible risks that go along with general or local anaesthesia.

After this first visit you will get the appointment for the surgery. The time between the two visits is very important for you to consider your decision. Here is some support to help you with your decision:

You have to sit back and think and rethink:

If you are sterilized you will not be able to become pregnant any more. Do you really want this? Here is some food for thought:

- ☐ Will I feel like less of a woman if I am sterile?
- ☐ Is my partner in favour of my decision to have a tubal ligation?
- ☐ Is my partner aware of the fact that we cannot have any children or any more children together?
- ☐ Have I thought about other possible methods of contraception, which are less risky and not as final? (e.g. vasectomy, IUD)
- ☐ Is there a possibility that my partner could change his mind and suddenly want to have another child with me?
- ☐ Is there a possibility that I might break up with my partner, meet somebody else and want to have a child with him or her?

Tubal ligation is not the right contraceptive method for you if you're changing partners. You still need condoms and spermicides to protect yourself from sexually transmitted infections and HIV.

Take some time to think about these questions. Discuss them with your partner and be really sure you still want the tubal ligation before you go for it!

Regret. Better to be sure than sorry!
Studies have shown that regret happens in 5% of cases. Here are the most common reasons why women regret their decision and contact their physicians to get a reversal. Could that happen to you as well?

Read this and check your own decision one more time:

- ☐ I was too young (under 30).
- ☐ I had young children, and now that they are grown we want another child.
- ☐ It is not going well in our relationship.
- ☐ I did not get enough information about it in the first place.
- ☐ I was pushed into it by my partner.
- ☐ I do not feel like a real woman any more.
- ☐ I found a new love and want a child with my new partner.
- ☐ My financial situation has improved and I can afford more children.

Some words about the surgery itself
There are three kinds of procedures:

1. Operating through a very small incision in the bellybutton. The procedure is called laparoscopy or band-aid surgery. It can be performed under local anaesthesia in some cases.

2. Operating through a larger incision in your belly. The procedure is called laparotomy. This also can be performed under local anaesthesia in some cases. It is less common, but often used when a tubal ligation is requested shortly after delivering a baby.

3. Operating through the vagina. This is called colpotomy and is hardly performed in North America.

The recovery period following a laparotomy is longer compared to a laparoscopy. The choice of the method depends on the physician and timing of the surgery.

Precautions after surgery

- No sports or physical strain for at least seven days after the surgery.
- If intense pain and high fever occur, contact your physician immediately.
- No restrictions on intercourse. Other than vasectomy, where there is a waiting period of three months, this method offers safe contraception from day one after surgery.

**A TUBAL LIGATION IS CONSIDERED PERMANENT
BECAUSE A REVERSAL IS DIFFICULT, COSTLY
AND NOT ALWAYS SUCCESSFUL.**

(?) If I ever regret the tubal ligation, is there a chance to reverse the procedure and become fertile again?

Yes, there is a chance. But it is much more complicated than the tubal ligation itself and it is very expensive. The probability of pregnancy following tubal ligation reversal is between 52 - 90%. Whether a reversal surgery is successful or not depends on how the surgery was first done and of course on the skills of the surgeon.

(?) Does it affect my desire, my ability to make love?

No. Think of the tubal ligation as a mechanical interruption of the transportation route of the eggs. The fact that the eggs cannot travel to the uterus has no effect on your hormones, cycles, periods, desire, lovemaking or ability to reach orgasm. Many women enjoy the freedom they feel after the procedure because they do not have to worry about contraception any more.

(?) Does it affect my periods?

Some women have reported changes in their cycles. This fact, however, could not be proven in studies.

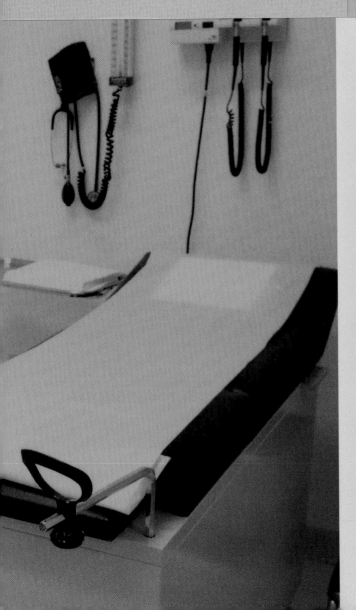

TROUBLESHOOTING

After the procedure there might be some reactions that cause discomfort. The most common are...

Pain at the site of the surgery	⚠
Bleeding	⚠
Nausea and light headedness (after the general anaesthesia)	⚠
Haematoma	⚠
Infection	⚠

Studies are ongoing to find out about the long-term complications of tubal ligation. Ectopic pregnancies (a pregnancy at the wrong place, meaning outside the uterus) are more likely to occur in women who have had a tubal ligation. If signs of pregnancy start showing you should contact your physician immediately.

VASECTOMY DISCONNECTION THE MALE WAY

What is vasectomy all about?
The surgery blocks the vas deferens (sperm duct) and prevents sperm from entering the ejaculate. The man can still ejaculate when reaching orgasm but the fluid, which leaves the penis during ejaculation, does not contain any sperm. The man is infertile and cannot make a woman pregnant any more. A vasectomy is considered permanent because a reversal is difficult and costly.

What makes the method so special?
- It is the most effective method of contraception controlled by the male partner (apart from abstinence).
- It is an easy procedure with very few known side effects.
- It is a permanent method.
- It is a good alternative if the female partner cannot use hormonal methods or the IUD.
- It relieves the woman from the contraceptive burden.

Does it protect against sexually transmitted infections and HIV?
No

How effective is vasectomy in preventing unintended pregnancy?
Pregnancy rate following vasectomy is 0-2.2%. Within three months after the procedure there is a risk of "recanalization," the disconnected vas deferens grows back together again. This happens in 2.6% of cases.

How do I get it?
You have to discuss this decision with your partner. You have to see a urologist or go to a family planning clinic. The physician will examine you and will find out whether you are a candidate for this procedure. After the procedure there is a three-month period during which time you can still have sperm in your ejaculate. Until you have your follow-up visit you have to use another form of contraception.

How much does it cost?
Usually covered by insurance. Additional costs when performed in a private practice vary from $75-200.

Possible problems
Certain discomforts like swelling following surgery. The biggest problem is regret. You have to really think about it and the consequences, and keep in mind that it is more or less permanent. The reversal does not always work out. Think and discuss with your partner!

WHAT IS VASECTOMY ALL ABOUT?

Vasectomy is also referred to as male sterilization. To be or to become sterile means that you cannot reproduce any more. The surgery blocks the right and left vas deferens to prevent the journey of the sperm into the ejaculate (fluid which leaves the penis during ejaculation). The man can still ejaculate but there is no more sperm in the ejaculate. He cannot make a woman pregnant any more. It is considered a permanent method of contraception chosen mostly by men who have completed their families because it is very difficult and costly to reverse the surgery.

How does vasectomy work?

You remember our anatomy chapter in the beginning of the book? It takes sperm around 70 days to mature. The mature sperm finally reaches the vas deferens. Sperm is stored in the vas deferens until ejaculation occurs. During ejaculation, sperm and liquid from the seminal vesicles make a mix that is called semen. When the vas deferens is cut sperm cannot get into the ejaculate. There are different techniques to do this and your physician will tell you about the choices you have.

How effective is vasectomy in preventing unintended pregnancy?

Pregnancy rates following vasectomy vary from 0 to 2.2%. It is, apart from female sterilization (called tubal ligation) and of course abstinence (no intercourse), the safest method of contraception. Now you might ask why a failure rate is still possible? The answer is simple. After the procedure there is a possibility that the testicular side of the vas finds its way and reaches the distant part of the vas (which was disconnected before). This complication is called recanalization (a communication recurs between the two ends of the vas). A recanalization can happen within the first three months after surgery in 2.6% of cases. This is why we recommend the use of a backup method between the time of surgery and the check-up visit three months later.

Does vasectomy protect against sexually transmitted infections and HIV?

No, it does not protect against sexually transmitted infections and HIV. Everything we have discussed in Chapter 2 on safer sex applies to sex partners who have chosen a vasectomy. The exchange of body fluids during intercourse makes bacterial and viral infections possible. The fact, for example, that there is no sperm in the ejaculate after a vasectomy was performed does not mean that there is a lower risk of infecting the female partner with an STI or HIV. A condom and spermicide protect you. Practice safer sex and use double protection!

Vasectomy is a good choice for you, if:

- you and your partner are sure that you do not want to have more or any children at all.
- you want a very effective, long-term method, which is safe, easy and not related to intercourse.
- you want to relieve your female partner from the contraceptive burden.
- your partner cannot use other methods which are reversible such as hormonal methods or the IUD.
- your partner is considering a tubal ligation (female sterilization). A vasectomy is easier and has less risk of side effects.

Vasectomy is not a good choice for you, if:

- you are not sure that you want permanent contraception.
- there is any possibility that you may regret this decision.

What to expect when getting a vasectomy?

First of all the physician who will perform the procedure will ask you a few questions. Please read the following paragraph to be prepared for some of them. It is very important to be absolutely sure that you want it done because it is a method of no return!

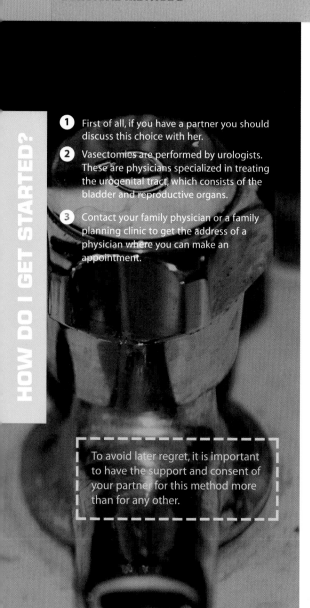

1 First of all, if you have a partner you should discuss this choice with her.

2 Vasectomies are performed by urologists. These are physicians specialized in treating the urogenital tract, which consists of the bladder and reproductive organs.

3 Contact your family physician or a family planning clinic to get the address of a physician where you can make an appointment.

To avoid later regret, it is important to have the support and consent of your partner for this method more than for any other.

Second, you will be examined to find out whether this procedure can be done.

After this first visit you will get the appointment for the vasectomy along with instructions how to prepare yourself for the surgery. The time between the two visits is very important to rethink your decision. Here is some support to help you with your decision:

You have to sit back and think and rethink:
After a vasectomy you will not be able to make babies. That is it, finished. Do you really want this? Here is some food for thought:

☐ Will I feel like less of a man if I am sterile?
☐ Is my partner in favour of my decision to have a vasectomy?
☐ Is my partner aware of the fact that we cannot have any children or any more children together?
☐ Is there a possibility that my female partner might change her mind and all of a sudden want to have another child with me?
☐ Is there a possibility that I could break up with my partner, meet another woman and want to have a child with her?

If you do not have a steady partner and you consider a vasectomy to protect yourself from becoming a father against your will, keep the following in mind:

• Women do not necessarily believe the man when he says: "You don't need a contraceptive because I had a vasectomy." The woman has no way of verifying this. She will probably insist on another contraceptive.

• Vasectomy is not the right contraceptive method if you want worry-free sex while you're changing partners. You still need a condom to protect yourself and your partner from sexually transmitted infections and HIV.

Take some time and think about these questions. Discuss them with your partner and be really sure you still want the vasectomy before you go for it!

Regret. Better to be sure than sorry!

Here are the most common reasons why men regret their decision and contact their physicians to get a reversal: Could that happen to you as well? Studies have shown that it happens in 5% of all cases. Read this and check your own decision one more time:

- ☐ I was too young (under 30).
- ☐ I had young children, and now that they are grown we want another child.
- ☐ It is not going well in our relationship.
- ☐ I did not get enough information.
- ☐ I was pushed into it by my partner.
- ☐ I do not feel like a real man any more.
- ☐ I found a new love and want a child with her.
- ☐ My financial situation has improved and I can afford more children.

Some words about the surgery itself

There are two ways to perform it:

1. The conventional way
   The skin of the scrotum is cut with a scalpel, the vas deferens is cut and 1.5 cm on each end of the vas is removed. The open ends are sealed along with the incision in the scrotum.

2. The no-scalpel vasectomy
   In this method a tiny cut using a puncture instead of a scalpel is made to go into the scrotum to cut the vas deferens.

Both procedures are performed under local anaesthesia. After the procedure you can go home. The no-scalpel method is associated with fewer complications than the conventional method.

Precautions after surgery

- No sports or physical strain for seven days after the surgery.
- No intercourse for five days.
- If strong pain and high fever occur, contact your physician immediately.
- Use another method of contraception for three months following surgery. There still might be sperm in your ejaculate. It takes about 15 ejaculations until the tubes are cleared of sperm. After this period you have to go for a check-up. A sperm count in the laboratory finds out whether your ejaculate is sperm-free and the vasectomy was a success.

The 1998 Canadian Contraception Study revealed that:	
14%	of respondents in the study used the method
>	since 1995 vasectomy has been more popular than tubal ligation

VASECTOMY IS NOT THE RIGHT CONTRACEPTIVE METHOD IF YOU WANT WORRY-FREE SEX WHILE YOU'RE CHANGING PARTNERS.

If I ever regret the vasectomy, is there a chance to reverse the procedure and become fertile again?

Yes, there is a chance. But, of course it's a hassle and the chances become slimmer the more time passes after the procedure. Here is a table to tell you what to expect.

PROBABILITY OF PREGNANCY FOLLOWING VASECTOMY REVERSAL

Time since vasectomy	Sperm in the semen (%)	Pregnancy (%)
Less than 3 years	97	76
3-8 years	88	53
9-14 years	79	44
More than 14 years	71	30

 Do I still produce sperm?

Yes. But since it cannot get out, the body absorbs it.

 Does it affect my desire, my ability to make love?

No. Think of the vasectomy as a mechanical interruption of a canal that transports sperm. This canal has nothing to do with sexual desire, ejaculation, or getting an erection. The man will still ejaculate but there won't be any more sperm in the ejaculate. It looks the same, though. Many couples even report an improved sex life because they do not have to worry about pregnancy any more. And it frees the woman from looking after contraception.

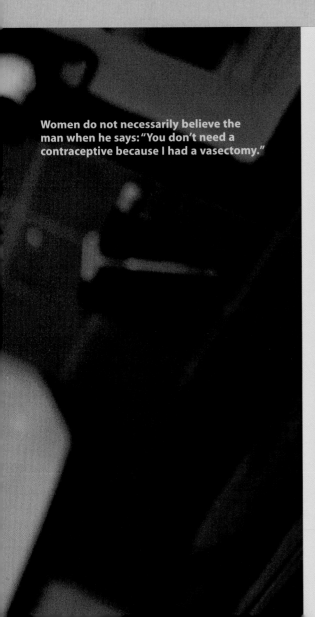

Women do not necessarily believe the man when he says: "You don't need a contraceptive because I had a vasectomy."

TROUBLESHOOTING

After the procedure there might be some reactions that cause discomfort. The most common are...

Pain at the site of the surgery	⚠
Swelling	⚠
Dizziness during the surgery	⚠
Haematoma (1-10%)	⚠
Infection (0.4-1%)	⚠

Studies are ongoing to find out about any long-term complications from a vasectomy. There have been concerns that a vasectomy might increase the risk of getting a cardiovascular disease, cancer of the testes and the prostate. It was proven in studies that there is no connection between vasectomy and cardiovascular disease nor cancer of the prostate.

In the 1998 Canadian Contraception Study, natural methods (including no sex at all) were used by 22% of respondents.

This chapter is about the following methods:

Abstinence

Withdrawal

Fertility Awareness

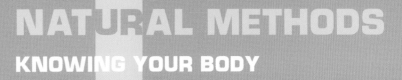

NATURAL METHODS
KNOWING YOUR BODY

"Natural" contraception means that there are no medications involved. The effectiveness of the methods in this chapter depends entirely on your and your partner's skills and talent! All natural methods depend on cooperation between partners and they are basically the cheapest methods in the world.

If you get serious about any of the following methods, you and your partner will benefit from them in many ways. They help you to better understand your bodies and maybe even your relationship!

The following information should help you to find out whether you are ready for this! For natural methods to work, you have to:

- Understand your body.
- Understand how fertilization works.
- Understand the female cycle.

And the most important thing: You have to discipline yourself and you need to have a partner who also supports the method and understands what it's all about.

This is not for the spontaneous amongst you! If spontaneity is key for you in your sex life please forget about natural methods of contraception. They are definitely not for you!

ABSTINENCE

What is abstinence all about?

The penis does not enter the vagina; in fact the penis does not even get close to the vagina. Abstinence also means that all sexual activities that lead to an exchange of body fluids are to be avoided.

What makes abstinence so special?

- Both partners have to talk and they have to agree on abstinence and what it means to their partnership.
- Abstinence encourages the use of other pleasuring techniques which might enrich the sexual relationship.
- It is a great method for the beginning stage of a relationship to test understanding and feelings for each other.
- Used in combination with fertility awareness methods.

Does it protect against sexually transmitted infections and HIV?

Yes. By avoiding skin to skin contact in the genital area and the mouth and the exchange of body fluids such as semen, blood, saliva and vaginal fluid. Abstinence is the most effective method in preventing pregnancy, STIs and HIV.

How effective is abstinence in preventing unintended pregnancy?

It is the most effective method on earth.

How do I get it?

It is free and available to everybody. You have to talk to your partner about it. It is very important that both of you agree to stay abstinent.

How much does it cost?

Nothing, just will power and consistency.

Possible problems

You and your partner have a different understanding of what abstinence is. Another problem is when you suddenly change your mind in the middle of sex play. Always have a condom with spermicide handy as a standby!

WHAT IS ABSTINENCE ALL ABOUT?

The word abstinence is used in many different contexts, e.g. abstinence from drugs, from alcohol. People choose abstinence for two reasons. They want to avoid pregnancy and/or infection with an STI or HIV. In the context of contraception and prevention of STIs, abstinence means:

- No intercourse.
- No sexual practice which might lead to an exchange of body fluids.
- No skin to skin contact in the genital area.
- No oral contact with the genitals.

Note: Some couples who are not at risk for STIs choose abstinence simply to avoid pregnancy. In that case, abstinence allows for a wide range of sexual expressions which may include the exchange of body fluids with only one exception: sperm.

How does abstinence work?

The penis does not enter the vagina and there is no exchange of body fluids such as:

- Pre-ejaculatory fluid
- Semen
- Secretion from the vagina
- Blood

Strictly speaking the penis should not get anywhere near the vagina. As mentioned in previous chapters, sperm has the ability to find its way into the vagina if ejaculation takes place at the entrance of the vagina. When practicing oral sex you have to be aware of the fact that mouth-vulva and mouth-penis contact can lead to a sexually transmitted infection. There are also certain STIs like HPV and herpes, which spread by skin to skin contact.

You might ask yourself: Isn't abstinence boring?

Well, not really. There are many ways to express love and desire other than intercourse. You might want to find out about pleasuring techniques that are allowed when using abstinence as a method. Here are some to give you an idea that intercourse is really only a small part of the fun!

- Kissing
- Hugging
- Masturbating
- Massaging
- Rubbing
- Looking at erotic material
- Breast / nipple stimulation

Do not let yourself be talked into intercourse by your friends or by your partner if you do not feel ready for it. It might be a good idea to wait for someone very special. It is your choice and it's your body. You are the boss!

By the way, here are some interesting findings of a survey. They say that the best things are worth waiting for. This very much applies to sex. Read how "the first time" turned out to be pretty disappointing for many:

**1999 Global Sex Survey:
FIRST TIME SEX**

Globally, almost 3 in 10 (29%) sexually active young people were disappointed by first sex, 17% found it much better than expected.

How effective is abstinence in preventing unintended pregnancy?

This is the most effective method of contraception on earth!

A word of caution: There is a chance that you might get carried away when you are intimate with your partner. In a moment of passion you might want to have intercourse. In that case it's handy to have a barrier method with you - just in case! It keeps you out of trouble in the long run. If you have no protection at all the last option is emergency contraception (Chapter 8). And: abstinence from drugs and alcohol helps you to keep control.

Does abstinence protect against sexually transmitted infections?

If you make sure that there is absolutely no exchange of body fluids, abstinence does protect you against STIs and HIV.

How popular is abstinence in Canada?

In the 1998 Canadian Contraception Study, abstinence was used by 14% of respondents. This figure includes the respondents who practice abstinence because they have no partner.

Abstinence is a good choice for you, if:

- you have not found the right partner yet.
- you are not sure about the state of your relationship.
- you are not sure about your partner.
- you want the safest contraceptive method on earth.
- you want to be protected against STIs and HIV.
- you do not want to make an appointment with your doctor.
- you want a method of contraception that guarantees no side effects.
- you like it "natural."

Abstinence is not for you, if:

- you are not sure about this choice.
- your partner is against it.
- you get lots of pressure from your partner or your peers to have sex and you are not sure you can stay firm in your decision to practice abstinence.

What to expect?

Like everything in life, your relationship might change and both of you might want to have intercourse. Then you have to consider another method of contraception and protection against STIs and HIV. To be on the safe side you might want to have condoms and spermicide with you in case you change your mind in the middle of sex play.

Where do I get it?

No consultation, no prescription needed! You have to talk to your partner about it. It is very important that both of you support this method. Imagine your partner tries to talk you into intercourse every time you make love. Then it is just a matter of time before the method fails.

**1999 Global Sex Survey:
WHY PEOPLE CHOSE TO WAIT**

The reasons for abstinence among the 1,400 respondents who were not sexually active yet, are:
47% do not feel ready yet.
27% feel ready, but did not meet the right partner yet.
9% lack of opportunity.
5% scared of discomfort/pain.
3% scared to not be good at it.
3% partner not ready yet.

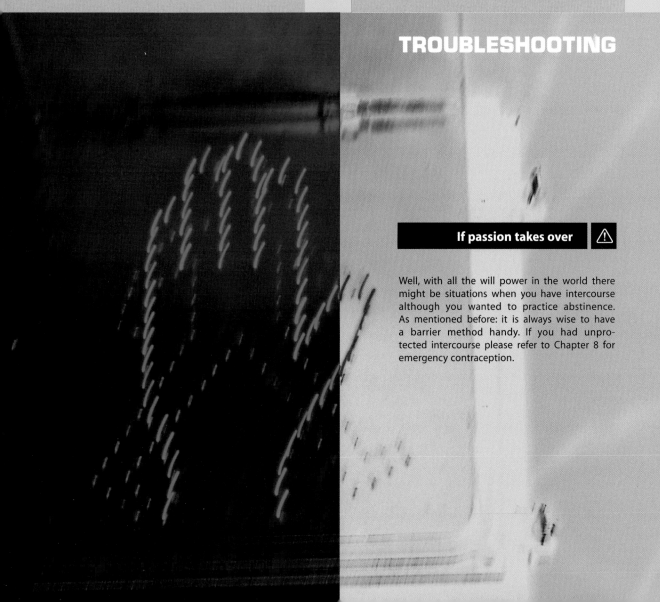

TROUBLESHOOTING

If passion takes over ⚠

Well, with all the will power in the world there might be situations when you have intercourse although you wanted to practice abstinence. As mentioned before: it is always wise to have a barrier method handy. If you had unprotected intercourse please refer to Chapter 8 for emergency contraception.

WITHDRAWAL

What is withdrawal all about?
The male partner withdraws the penis from the vagina before ejaculation.

How effective is withdrawal in preventing unintended pregnancy?
It is not very effective because there might be sperm in the pre-ejaculate, which can lead to fertilization. Studies have shown a failure rate of 19% in typical users and 4 % in perfect users.

Does it protect against sexually transmitted infections and HIV?
No

How much does it cost?
Nothing, just some self-discipline and practice.

How do I get it?
You have to talk to your partner about it. We also highly recommend that you practice with a condom and spermicide first, especially if you and your partner have not been together long.

What makes withdrawal so special?
- It requires self-control.
- It needs practice.
- It requires that both partners cooperate.
- It is a great method when no other methods are available (better than nothing!).

Possible problems
- Inexperience of both partners.
- No control over time of ejaculation.
- Frustration because of the interruption.

WHAT IS WITHDRAWAL ALL ABOUT?

Withdrawal is a method that is called by its Latin name "coitus interruptus." This term means interrupted intercourse. You stop the action before it's finished! It does not offer great protection against pregnancy but it is better than no method at all! When you get stuck in a situation when you and your lover want to have sex and you have no method handy...use this one!

How does withdrawal work?
The man draws the penis out of the vagina and away from the entrance of the vagina before ejaculation occurs. This way he prevents sperm from entering the vagina and sperm cannot meet the female egg for fertilization.

How effective is withdrawal in preventing unintended pregnancy?
There are two reasons why this method is unreliable:

1. This method is entirely based on will power and practice.
2. There might be sperm in the pre-ejaculate of the erect penis, which gets into the vagina before the penis is withdrawn.

Some studies have shown a failure rate of 4% during the first year of use among users who applied the method perfectly. Typical use had a failure rate of 19%.

Does it protect against sexually transmitted infections and HIV?
No. Withdrawal only prevents the semen from getting into the vagina. The man is not protected because the penis is exposed to the fluids inside the vagina during intercourse. The woman is not protected because the vagina is exposed to the pre-ejaculate, which can lead to sexually transmitted or HIV infections.

How popular is withdrawal in Canada?
In the 1998 Canadian Contraception Study, withdrawal was used by 6% of respondents. Six times as many Canadian women rely on withdrawal as currently use the IUD.

Withdrawal is a good choice for you, if:

- both you and your partner are free of STIs and HIV.
- you are mutually faithful to each other and you can trust each other.
- the male partner is used to this method and has not experienced any failures.
- you both agree on this method and cooperate accordingly.
- you can live with a certain risk of getting pregnant.

Withdrawal is not for you, if:

- there is an STI/HIV risk.
- you are looking for a long-term, effective method.
- you and your partner get carried away easily during lovemaking.
- the male partner cannot anticipate orgasm and ejaculation.
- you had previous failure with this method.
- you consider withdrawal to be an interruption of lovemaking.

Where do I get it?
You have to talk to your partner about it. It is very important that both of you support this method. Withdrawal can be frustrating at times because it interrupts the sex play.

What to expect?
Like everything in life, your relationship might change and both of you may want to stop the withdrawal technique. Then you have to consider another method of contraception and protection against STIs and HIV. To be on the safe side you might want to have condoms or other barrier methods with you in case you change your mind while having sex.

TROUBLESHOOTING

The effectiveness of this method is highly dependent upon the cooperation of both partners.

Pulled out too late

This is the most common reason for failure of this method! Don't panic! Read Chapter 8 on emergency contraception.

Frustration

This might be an issue. The withdrawal method needs practice to be acceptable for both partners. Both of you have to learn to continue pleasuring each other after the penis has left the vagina in order not to make the withdrawal a break-off point during your sex play.

Inexperience

A word of caution to the woman: If you are in a new relationship and your partner says that he is an expert in withdrawal, you should use a condom and spermicide anyway. You have to get used to each other and to each other's reactions first. To rely on the withdrawal method at the start of a new relationship is like playing with fire.

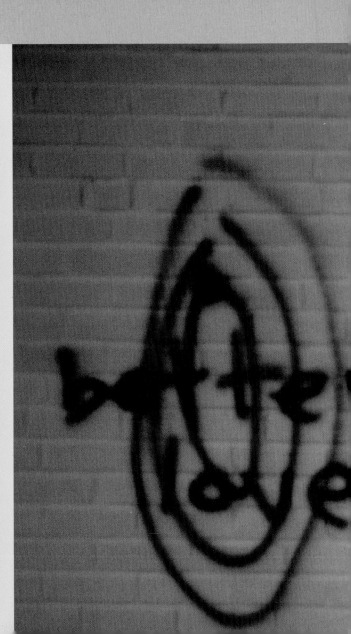

Do you know why withdrawal is also called the "basketball technique?"

He dribbles before he shoots!!!

FERTILITY AWARENESS

What is fertility awareness all about?
The woman keeps track of her monthly cycle by taking her temperature, by checking the vaginal mucus or by tracking other information in a calendar. The idea behind all these methods is to find a pattern behind the individual cycle to predict when the woman is fertile. During the fertile period the partners have to abstain from intercourse or use another method of contraception.

What makes the method so special?
- It requires knowledge and self-control.
- It helps you understand your body and your cycle.
- It requires that both partners cooperate.
- It can also be used to actually plan a pregnancy when you are ready for it.

Does it protect against sexually transmitted infections and HIV?
No

How effective is fertility awareness in preventing unintended pregnancy?
It is not very effective. You and your partner should be willing to accept a pregnancy. Studies have shown pregnancy rates of up to 20% in the first year of use.

How do I get it?
You have to talk to your partner about it. This method needs the cooperation of your partner. You also have to get more information than this book provides.

How much does it cost?
Nothing, just self-discipline, knowledge and time to keep track of fertility data every day.

Possible problems
Lack of knowledge and events which disturb your cycle (illness, stress, peri-menopause, adolescence).

WHAT IS FERTILITY AWARENESS ALL ABOUT?

Fertility awareness is used as a contraceptive method and as a method for those who want to plan a pregnancy. In this book we will concentrate on its use as a contraceptive. Fertility awareness requires knowledge and skills we are not able to address in detail. We recommend further reading. You should contact the closest Planned Parenthood office, a family planning clinic, or Serena, an organization that teaches and provides information on natural family planning. They can provide you with detailed information on fertility awareness methods. Please refer to the address section.

There are various techniques used to practice fertility awareness. The idea behind all these techniques is to determine the fertile days in the individual's cycle. With the knowledge of this fertile time period, intercourse can be avoided or another method of contraception used.

How does fertility awareness work?

You have to learn when your fertile days are and abstain from intercourse or use other methods of contraception during this fertile period. The method requires knowledge and discipline.

What are the principles of fertility awareness?

1. The period starts 14 days after the egg is released from an ovary (ovulation).
2. The female egg lives for 1 day only.
3. Sperm can survive a couple of days in the woman's body and can fertilze an egg during this time.
4. Fertilization can therefore happen days after intercourse.
5. The "safe days" during which a woman cannot conceive are from day 2 after ovulation until the new period starts.

Keeping these principles in mind, guess what the big challenge is? To find out when ovulation happens during the cycle. Here are the methods to determine the fertile days:

Calendar Rhythm Method Idea behind this method: When you keep track of your cycle using a calendar for a few months, you will begin to see a pattern developing. This pattern allows you to determine a time frame when ovulation occurs each month. You simply calculate: The shortest cycle minus 19 days (example: 26 - 19 = 7), the longest cycle minus 10 days (example: 32 - 10 = 22). This calculation gives you a window from day 7 to day 22 during which time you must abstain from vaginal intercourse or use a contraceptive.

Basal Body Temperature Method Idea behind this method: Body temperature rises on the day of ovulation and stays 0.5 degrees higher two days after ovulation. The woman has to keep track of her temperature and mark the readings in a calendar. You will see a pattern developing.

Ovulation or Billings Method Idea behind this method: One day before, during and one day after ovulation the mucus in front of the cervix becomes slippery, elastic and clear. The woman has to insert her fingers in the vagina and check the quality of the mucus to determine the time of ovulation.

Symptothermal Method Idea behind this method: It uses the principles of the first two methods. Using a calendar, the woman keeps track of her temperature and the changes of the vaginal mucus.

Ovulation Predictor Kits There are kits available in the drugstore, which help to predict when ovulation occurs. They test the urine for the presence of a hormone, which shows that ovulation will occur shortly. These are generally used by women who want to conceive. They are also a great tool to help you understand your cycle.

Breast-feeding   Idea behind it: Breast-feeding suppresses ovulation. Breast-feeding protects against pregnancy for a period of 6 months after the birth of the baby provided:

- The woman has not yet had her first period since giving birth.
- The woman breast-feeds the baby regularly and does not use formula in addition to the breast milk.
- There is no more than 4 hours between feeds.

This method has been shown to be effective in 98% of all cases.

How effective are fertility awareness methods in preventing unintended pregnancy?
Not very effective. Studies have shown that 20% of users became pregnant within the first year of using one of the fertility awareness methods.

The big exception is breast-feeding which has a very low failure rate of 2% provided you respect the above conditions.

Do fertility awareness methods protect against sexually transmitted infections?
No. Practice safer sex: Use a condom and spermicide to get double protection against STIs and HIV.

Fertility awareness is a good choice for you, if:

- you are willing to invest some time and effort to become familiar with a fertility awareness method.
- you and your partner are willing to respect your fertile days (meaning: no intercourse, otherwise another contraceptive method must be used).
- you like it natural.
- you enjoy learning more about your body and you enjoy "listening" to your body.
- you want a method of contraception with a guarantee of no side effects.

Fertility awareness is not for you, if:

- you need protection against STIs and HIV.
- your partner is against it and does not want to cooperate.
- you are not willing to invest time to become familiar with a method.
- routine is not your cup of tea.

What do I have to expect?
Certain frustrations and many questions. For example, if you become ill the whole tracking system will no longer give the right information. The methods only work when you are healthy and your periods are more or less regular. If you used a hormonal method before, you have to wait a few months until your natural cycle returns before you start with fertility awareness.

It is basically only recommended when you and your partner can accept the failure of this method!

Where do I get it?
You have to talk to your partner about it. It is very important that both of you support fertility awareness as a contraceptive method. The best idea is to consult Planned Parenthood, a family planning clinic, or Serena.

The 1998 Canadian Contraception Study revealed that:	
2%	of respondents used fertility awareness

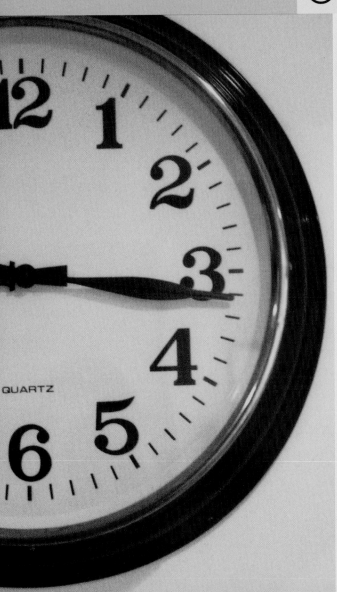

QUARTZ

TROUBLESHOOTING

The effectiveness of this method is highly dependent upon the cooperation of both partners. The woman's job is to keep track of her fertile and infertile days, while the man has to respect her fertile days and accept no intercourse or the use of another contraceptive method during this time. Possible problems are...

| Stress and illness | |

Stress and illness can change the menstrual cycle. You will have to use another method of contraception until the cycle becomes regular again.

| Age | |

Fertility awareness does not work for adolescents because the cycles are not established and regular. Women in peri-menopause also should not rely on this method because the cycles often become irregular before they stop altogether.

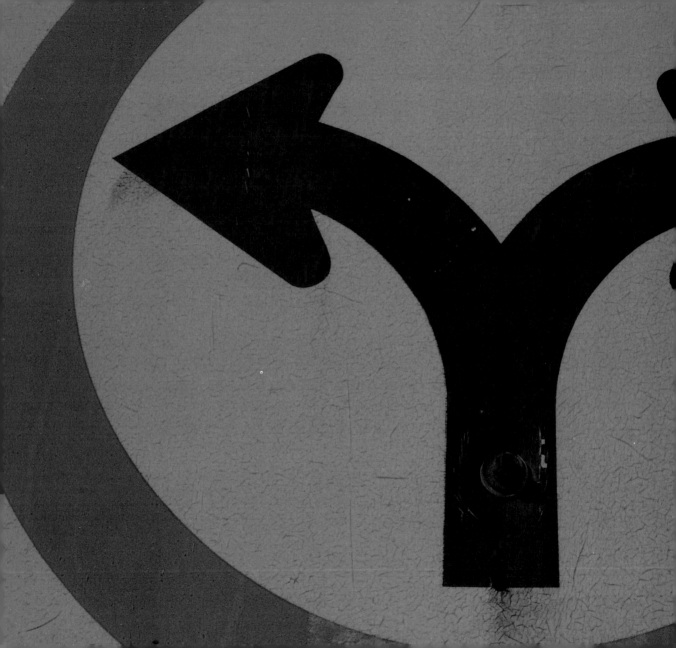

INTRAUTERINE METHOD

FOR THE LONG-TERM RELATIONSHIP

This method is unique in comparison to all other methods and devices. The IUD looks like a barrier method but it stands apart from all the methods discussed in Chapter 4. The contraceptive action is based on a chemical reaction. Furthermore, while other barrier methods have to be inserted and removed before and after intercourse, the IUD can stay in the uterus for many years.

IUD **INTRAUTERINE DEVICE**

What is the IUD all about?
A plastic, T-shaped device with a copper wire. A physician performs the placement of the device in the uterus. The copper wire changes the chemistry in the uterus and destroys sperm. It is a safe and effective contraceptive for women who have already given birth, who are at low risk of acquiring sexually transmitted infections and who want long-term contraception (5-8 years).

What makes the IUD so special?
- Independent from intercourse.
- Long-term contraception for up to 8 years.
- No negative impact on fertility after removal.
- Good choice for women who cannot use or do not want hormonal methods.
- No effect on breast milk.
- Good alternative to sterilization.
- Good for family spacing.
- Can be used as an emergency contraceptive up to 7 days after unprotected intercourse.

Does it protect against sexually transmitted infections and HIV?
No

How effective is the IUD in preventing unintended pregnancy?
98% effective.

How do I get it?
You have to see your family doctor, a gynaecologist or a family planning clinic. It usually requires two visits. First visit: a history is taken, followed by a physical exam and a testing for STIs. Second visit: the actual insertion of the IUD.

How much does it cost?
Between $50-150.

Possible problems
Pain and bleeding after the insertion. There is also an increased risk of pelvic inflammatory disease for a period of three months following the insertion or in the case of acquiring an STI.

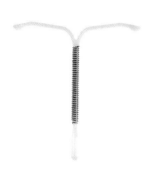

Actual size

WHAT IS THE IUD ALL ABOUT?

Intrauterine means inside the uterus. The arms of the IUD are flexible and gently rounded to help with insertion and removal. Insertion and removal is the job of a physician. A copper wire surrounds the T-shaped plastic frame. At the bottom of the IUD there is a polyethylene string. Because the shape of the device mirrors the shape of the uterus, it fits snugly in place without you feeling it.

The IUD is a very effective long-term method of contraception. It can stay in the uterus from 5-8 years. If the IUD is inserted during the late reproductive years of a woman (in her forties), it can be left in the uterus until menopause. The IUD is also used as an emergency contraceptive that can prevent ovulation within 7 days of unprotected intercourse. The IUD is a contraceptive for women who are not at risk for STIs and have a normal uterus.

Why is that so?

An exclusive relationship (one partner only) is an important condition simply because there is an increased risk of developing STIs and pelvic inflammatory disease (PID) when an IUD is in the uterus and the woman or her partner have more than just each other as sex partners.

How does the IUD work?

The copper wire surrounding the plastic frame creates a chemical environment in the uterus that is unfriendly towards sperm and eggs. The chemical reaction provoked by the copper inside the uterus also destroys sperm so that sperm has no chance to travel to the fallopian tubes and fertilization cannot take place.

How effective is the IUD in preventing unintended pregnancy?

This method is 98% effective. If 100 women use this method over a period of one year, two women may become pregnant.

Does the IUD protect against sexually transmitted infections and HIV?

No. The use of a male condom and spermicide is necessary to be protected. Practice safer sex: use double protection. The presence of a sexually transmitted infection while an IUD is in place dramatically increases the risk of pelvic inflammatory disease and thus the risk of infertility.

The 1998 Canadian Contraception Study revealed that:	
1%	of respondents in the study used the IUD

1 You need to make an appointment with your family doctor, a gynaecologist or at a family planning clinic. You should inquire about it when you ask for an appointment because not all physicians insert IUDs. The doctor will have to perform a medical exam, take your history, and ask questions about your sex life. (see page 28) It is very important to be frank in answering these questions. It is in your own best interest to find out together with your physician whether this is the right method for you. The IUD is really not a good idea if you are at an increased risk for sexually transmitted infections or you have already experienced an STI.

There are also certain health conditions that speak against the use of an IUD. Usually at the first visit you will be tested for possible infections or diseases.

2 At a second visit, after the results of the tests have arrived, the insertion will be done.

3 A follow-up visit after three months is a good idea. You will be able to ask questions and talk about possible effects that bother you. If everything goes well you should go back once a year for a check-up.

The IUD is an effective contraceptive method right away. From day one of insertion you are protected from unintended pregnancy. The insertion can be done anytime during your cycle. If you have just given birth you have to wait 4-6 weeks.

The IUD is also an effective emergency contraceptive. If it is inserted even as late as seven days after unprotected intercourse, it can prevent pregnancy (Chapter 8). After an abortion the IUD can be inserted immediately following the procedure.

The IUD is a good choice for you, if:

- you have a steady sexual partner (you are faithful to him, he is faithful to you).
- you want a long-term reliable method.
- you want to practice "family spacing."
- you have had failure with other methods in the past (you cannot remember to take a pill daily or you tend to forget to have barrier methods with you).
- you are breast-feeding (the IUD has no effect on breast milk).
- you have completed your family and seek an alternative to tubal ligation.
- you have a problem with hormonal methods.

The IUD is not for you, if:

- you are pregnant.
- you change sexual partners frequently.
- you have an infection or inflammation in your lower body parts.
- you suffer from diseases that weaken your immune system.
- you have bleeding from the vagina that is not related to your period.
- you have allergies to the material the IUDs are made of.

How does the insertion work?

The insertion by an experienced physician should not cause more than slight discomfort. Before inserting the IUD, your doctor will gently slide a speculum into the vagina in order to make room for the fitting. After that the depth of the uterus will be measured to find the correct position for the IUD. Using an insertion tube the doctor will gently slide it through your vagina and into your uterus. When it is in place the arm will open up and form the T-shape.

What IUDs are available in Canada?

Currently there are only two kinds available: Nova-T and GyneT. A new IUD containing a progestin will be introduced within the next two years.

THE IUD IS A CONTRACEPTIVE FOR WOMEN WHO ARE NOT AT RISK FOR SEXUALLY TRANSMITTED INFECTIONS AND HAVE A NORMAL UTERUS.

⑦ Does the IUD have an effect on my fertility?

No. Women who have had their IUDs removed have the same chance of becoming pregnant as women who never used the IUD at all.

⑦ Do I have to check the strings after each period?

No. You do not need to check the strings to make sure the IUD is still in place. This advice is outdated.

TROUBLESHOOTING

The IUD gets rejected and expelled

In the very rare event that you lose the IUD after insertion you have to see your doctor or go to a clinic right away.

Unscheduled bleeding

The IUD should not interfere with the normal menstrual cycle because it does not interfere with the hormones in your blood. However, in the rare event of unscheduled bleeding you should contact your physician or family planning clinic. Cramps and slight bleeding following the insertion of the IUD are normal.

Heavier menstrual bleeding and pain

Studies have shown that 5-15% of IUD users have the device removed after one year of use because they experience more pain and heavier bleeding during periods.

The partner feels the strings

Although the strings attached to the IUD are cut short after the insertion, it is possible that the male partner might feel the strings at the tip of his penis during intercourse. If that occurs talk to your physician about it.

Pelvic inflammatory disease (PID)

At one point there was a lot of talk about PID and IUDs. Recent studies have shown that PID is related to the exposure to sexually transmitted infections rather than to IUD use. In the first three months after the insertion of the device there is an increased risk of PID which is related to the insertion procedure and to the chemical reaction caused by the copper wire.

Pregnancy complications

In the unlikely event of a pregnancy with the IUD in place, your doctor should remove the device immediately. If not, there is a greater risk of losing the baby (spontaneous abortion) or having a delivery before the baby is fully grown. Birth defects have not been reported with an IUD in place. You might also want to turn to Chapter 8 where we explain the role of IUDs in emergency contraception.

Ectopic pregnancy

This is a pregnancy that happens out of place. The fetus grows somewhere other than in the uterus, most likely in the fallopian tubes. If you become pregnant with an IUD in place, there is a greater than normal chance that this could be an ectopic pregnancy. This causes considerable pain and is an emergency situation.

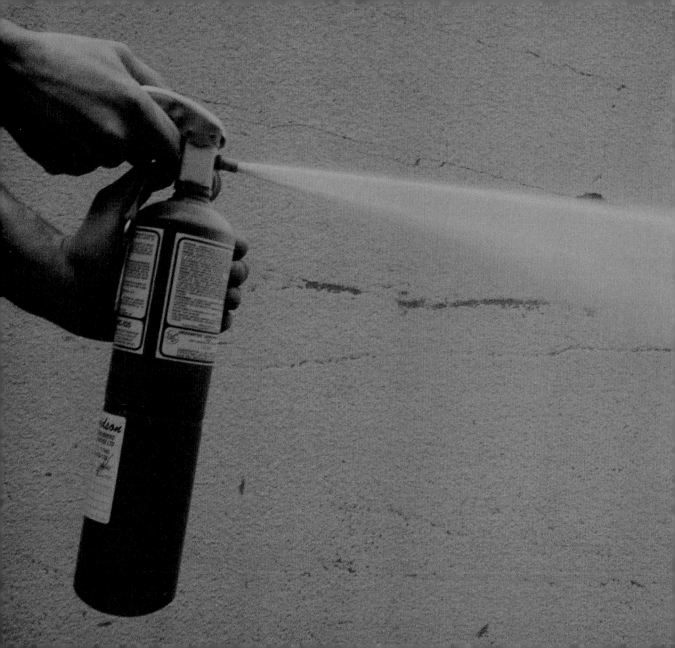

ALL ABOUT EMERGENCY CONTRACEPTION

You had sex and… in the heat of the moment… forgot all about contraception! Or - something went wrong with your barrier method, the diaphragm moved out of place, the condom slipped off… Well, those things happen in life and it's not the end of the world. However, taking a bath, using lots of soap, applying vaginal douche or just hoping that you won't get pregnant won't help.

EMERGENCY CONTRACEPTION

What is emergency contraception (EC) all about?

EC can be used to prevent pregnancy after unprotected intercourse or when a contraceptive method has failed or wasn't used correctly.

- The Emergency OC Method delays or prevents ovulation and works as late as 72 hours after unprotected intercourse.
- The IUD method creates a chemical environment in the uterus that is unfriendly to sperm and eggs. It works up to 7 days after unprotected intercourse.

What makes the method so special?

It is a simple and safe way to prevent pregnancy when something goes wrong with your contraceptive or you were forced into having sex provided you act fast enough and contact your physician or a clinic within 72 hours of unprotected intercourse.

Does it protect against sexually transmitted infections and HIV?

No

How effective is the Emergency OC in preventing unintended pregnancy?

The Emergency OC Method prevents 3 pregnancies out of 4.

How do I get it?

The Emergency OC Method: go to a community health centre, walk-in clinic, or call your family physician or gynaecologist and explain what happened. In most cases you can get a prescription over the phone. The sooner you take it, the greater the efficacy!

The IUD method: you have to make an appointment with your physician a.s.a.p. Make it clear that you need emergency contraception so that you get an appointment immediately. You can also go directly to a family planning clinic.

How much does it cost?

Costs vary greatly depending on method and where you get it from.

Possible problems

Nausea in 25%, vomiting in 6.2% of users of the Emergency OC Method.

WHAT IS EMERGENCY CONTRACEPTION ALL ABOUT?

There are two emergency contraceptive methods used in Canada:

1. The oral contraceptive method (OC): works within 72 hours of unprotected intercourse.
2. The intrauterine device method (IUD): works within 7 days of unprotected intercourse.

One of Canada's best kept health secrets

Emergency contraception is one of Canada's best kept health secrets and therefore seldom used. Its wider use could dramatically reduce unintended pregnancies and abortions.

EC is also referred to as post-coital contraception; the method is used after intercourse (=post-coital) as opposed to other methods which are used before or during intercourse. EC is also known as the "Morning after Pill." This is a bit misleading because this term only includes the oral contraceptive method and this method can actually be used even later than the "morning after." In fact, it works as late as 72 hours after intercourse, but studies show that the sooner you take it, the better the efficacy.

EC prevents pregnancy in the following situations:

- The condom comes off or breaks.
- Your diaphragm/cervical cap goes out of position during intercourse.
- You miscalculated your non-fertile days and didn't use contraception.
- You missed taking some oral contraceptive pills.
- You were forced into sex.
- You and your partner did not use any method at all.

How does the Emergency OC Method work?

The Emergency OC Method works the same way as an oral contraceptive works. After unprotected intercourse or after the failure or suspected failure of a method, you will get four combined oral contraceptive pills. Each tablet contains 250 mcg of the progestogen levonorgestrel and 50 mcg of the estrogen ethinyl estradiol. (It is also call "the Yuzpe method", named after the Canadian gynaecologist who developed it.) This is a higher dose than you would normally take when you take OCs as your daily method of contraception. It prevents or delays ovulation and saves you from getting pregnant. This method works up to 72 hours after intercourse. You have to take the first two pills no later than 72 hours after intercourse.

How effective is the Emergency OC Method in preventing unintended pregnancy?

The Emergency OC Method can prevent 3 pregnancies out of 4, which could be expected after one single act of unprotected intercourse, provided you take it no later than 72 hours after intercourse. However, your fertility depends on the time in the cycle when the emergency situation occurred. The days surrounding ovulation are the most "dangerous". Generally speaking there is a 25% chance of becoming pregnant when you've had unprotected sex or experienced contraceptive failure.

Does the Emergency OC Method protect against sexually transmitted infections and HIV?

No. If you had unprotected sex and are not sure about the health of your partner, you should take advantage of your emergency to visit your physician or family planning clinic not only to get emergency contraception but also to discuss STI testing. This especially applies to women who were forced into sex.

How popular is the Emergency OC Method in Canada?

There are no statistics available. Up until 1999, physicians were prescribing certain oral contraceptive pills and copper IUDs for emergency contraception because there was no specific emergency contraceptive available. In the fall of 1999 the Preven emergency contraceptive kit was introduced. This will make it easier to trace the use of this method in the future. A new emergency contraceptive, which contains only a progestin, is pending approval.

1. Read the instructions you received.

2. Immediately take two tablets with a glass of water.

3. Take the second set of two tablets exactly 12 hours later. This is a pretty strong dose for your body to take at once. You might feel a little sick.

4. If you have to vomit within one hour of taking the pills you will have to repeat the dose. The doctor might recommend a medication against sickness to avoid this problem.

5. You will start your period within 21 days after taking the pills.

TROUBLESHOOTING

Nausea

Nausea occurs in 25% of users, vomiting in 6.2% of cases. If you vomit within one hour of taking the tablets, you have to take the same dose again. Other effects might be irregular menstruation after use, breast tenderness, headache, abdominal pain and dizziness. These effects are due to a relatively high dose of hormones taken in a short period of time. These effects normally disappear within a couple of hours but might last up to two days.

No bleeding after taking the Emergency OC Method

In this case chances are that you are pregnant. Go to the pharmacy and buy a pregnancy test. (If you have the Preven EC kit, a pregnancy test is already included.) If you are pregnant see your doctor or family planning clinic again and discuss your options.

Serious side effects

Serious side effects such as blood clots, stroke and heart attack are extremely rare.

The IUD method, in the context of emergency contraception, has the same features that apply under "normal" circumstances. After insertion the IUD acts as a long-term contraceptive. It is mainly for women who cannot take hormones and who want a long-term and very effective contraceptive. For the IUD method please refer to Chapter 7.

The Emergency OC Method is a "one shot" method, which implies that you have to make a contraceptive choice after using it. In this chapter we concentrate on the Emergency OC Method.

Can any woman use the Emergency OC Method?
The answer is yes, almost any woman. There are only a few exceptions. Those are:

- You are already pregnant from a previous act of intercourse. However, if you use EC and you are already pregnant it will not cause harm to the pregnancy.
- You suffer from active thromboembolic disease.
- Your "emergency" situation occurred more than 72 hours ago. In this case the IUD might be a better choice because this method works even 7 days after unprotected intercourse. Read Chapter 7.
- If you haven't had your period for more than 4 weeks, your health care provider may suggest a pregnancy test before prescribing you this method.

Where do I get the Emergency OC Method?
You can go to a walk-in clinic or you can call your family physician, gynaecologist or family planning clinic and explain the situation. In some cases you don't even have to show up. If you have the name, address and phone number of your pharmacist, your physician might send the prescription directly to the pharmacist for you to pick up. You won't have to worry about an exam, your parents and embarrassing questions.

However, it is recommended that you see a physician. This is a good chance to ask him or her about contraception. Use this experience to think about contraception so you will not run into this panic again. A good idea is to ask your physician for an advance prescription. This is especially convenient if you are relying on barrier methods of contraception which have a higher probability of user failure!

For more information check out the website: **www.preven.com**

The 1998 Canadian Contraception Study revealed that

46%	of respondents knew that emergency contraception exists

THE EMERGENCY OC METHOD IS SIMPLE, EASY TO USE AND HAS MINIMAL MEDICAL RISK. THE EXPOSURE TO DRUGS IS SHORT AND SIDE EFFECTS DO NOT USUALLY LAST LONG.

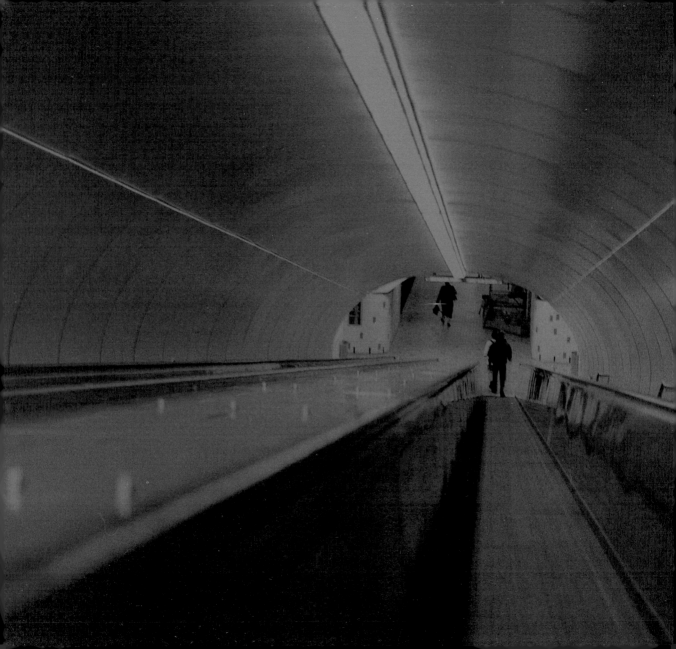

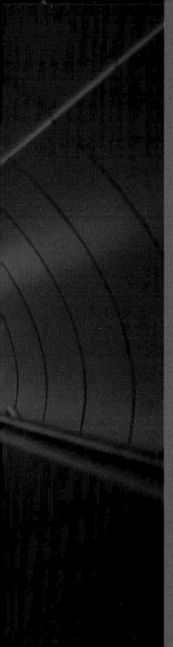

RETHINK AND ADJUST

CONTRACEPTION FOR THE PHASES OF YOUR LIFE

A woman can be fertile for over 30 years if we consider that the first period (menarche) is at age 12 and the last period (menopause) at around 50. Men can father children until very old age. It is one of the big health challenges in our lives to protect ourselves from unintended pregnancy and infections during this long period of fertile years! A contraceptive that suits you and your partner well when you are 20 might be out of the question when you are 40.

CATEGORIES OF METHODS: A CHAPTER OVERVIEW

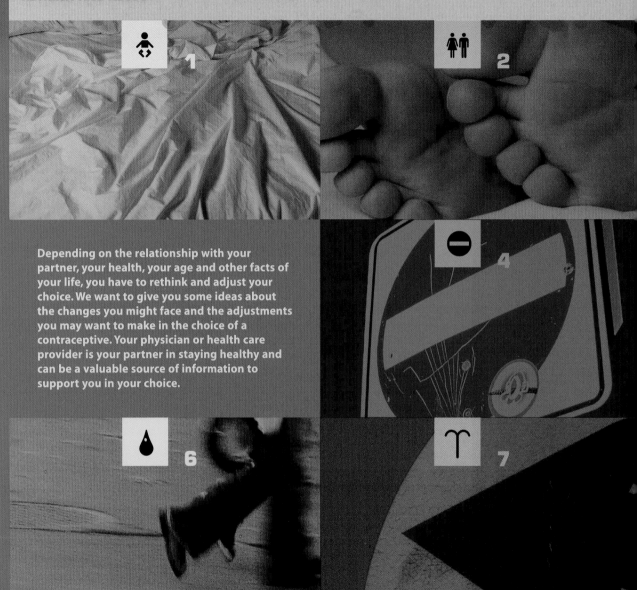

1

2

4

Depending on the relationship with your partner, your health, your age and other facts of your life, you have to rethink and adjust your choice. We want to give you some ideas about the changes you might face and the adjustments you may want to make in the choice of a contraceptive. Your physician or health care provider is your partner in staying healthy and can be a valuable source of information to support you in your choice.

6

7

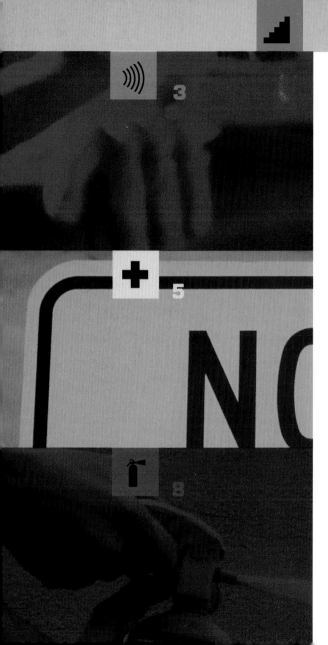

Adolescence

Your adolescent years are years of exploration and orientation. You will want to check out what sex is all about and you might have more than just one partner.

When you make your choice, think of the following:

You want a very effective method because a pregnancy is probably the last thing you desire and you want protection against STIs and HIV. You also want to preserve your fertility. Practice safer sex: use double protection.

In your adolescent years you have the highest chance of getting infected. HIV and AIDS can kill you. Other STIs, if not treated early, can lead to infertility in men and women. This could be very bad news if you plan to have a family later on. Use a condom (the male latex or the female condom) and a spermicide and you will be protected.

A good choice if you are healthy is to take the pill to protect yourself against pregnancy and to use a condom and a spermicide to protect you and your partner against STIs and HIV.

Hormonal methods used with condoms are the most effective methods. Refer to **Chapter 3** and Chapter 4 and discuss the choices with your health care provider and your partner. If you cannot take the pill, progestin-only methods are great, too.

One more thing about the pill: The pill is a great choice for healthy women. However, you have to follow the daily pill-taking schedule. You should also consider the pill as a long-term method of contraception. If you break up with your boyfriend you should not stop taking the pill. Why is that?

- The body has to adjust every time you start or stop the pill.
- You have to readjust every time to get back into the routine of taking the pill every day.

- The pill offers health benefits apart from being a very effective contraceptive.
- No sex doesn't mean that you should not take the pill. You might find another partner and you will be protected against pregnancy if you keep on taking the pill. Remember that until both of you have tested negative for sexually transmitted infections, you should use condoms and spermicides.

We do not want to discourage you from using the sponge, diaphragm and cap. The only problem with these methods is the high risk of failure. They also require more practice for correct and consistent use.

After giving birth

If you just gave birth you are facing many decisions. Do I want another child and when? Do I want to breast-feed my baby? We want to give you support for your decision in terms of contraception. Breast-feeding suppresses ovulation. Breast-feeding protects against pregnancy for a period of six months following the birth of the baby provided:

- The woman has not yet had her first period since giving birth.
- The woman breast-feeds the baby regularly and does not use formula in addition to the breast milk.
- There are no more than four hours between feeds.

IF YOU DO NOT MEET THESE CONDITIONS YOU CAN BECOME PREGNANT EVEN WHEN YOU ARE BREAST-FEEDING.

The IUD and progestin-only contraceptives are a good choice for women who have given birth and breast-feed because they do not affect the quality and quantity of breast milk. If you are not breast-feeding you can start taking the oral contraceptive pill 3-4 weeks after delivery. Some couples may consider a permanent method of contraception and choose tubal ligation or vasectomy. Barrier methods such as condoms and spermicides do not have any effect on your system and can be used any time. The diaphragm and cervical cap require refitting after giving birth.

After a known or suspected contraceptive failure

If you do not want to become pregnant you have to use emergency contraception. The Emergency OC Method works within 72 hours of unprotected intercourse and the IUD method works up to 7 days afterwards. Contact your health care provider immediately and refer to **Chapter 8**.

After an abortion

Most likely something went wrong with your contraceptive or you did not use any contraceptive at all. Depending on the stage of your life you may want to choose a more effective method after this experience. You have to ask yourself how it happened and how you can prevent it in the future.

- Did you or your partner fail in using a contraceptive method?
- Did the method fail?
- Did you use any contraceptive?

No matter what the answers to the above questions may be, you have to change something to avoid an unintended pregnancy in the future. If you want to have children in the future you should consider a hormonal method of contraception. If you do not want any more pregnancies, a long-term method (IUD, vasectomy, tubal ligation, implant) might be good for you.

You are a smoker

Stop smoking! If you are a woman and 35 years of age or older and do not want to or cannot stop smoking you should stop taking the oral contraceptive pill. The pill makes the dangerous habit of smoking even more dangerous. Stop smoking! If you like using hormonal contraception you can switch to any of the three progestin-only methods described in **Chapter 3**. You may also want to consider the IUD (Chapter 7). Guys among you: same thing! Stop smoking!

Approaching menopause

A woman in her late reproductive years is facing major changes in menopause. She may think about taking hormone replacement therapy to ease menopausal symptoms such as hot flushes, night sweats, vaginal dryness and to protect herself against cardiovascular disease and osteoporosis. In the years before menopause (menopause is considered when one year has passed since the last menstrual period) the cycles become irregular. What many women forget is that they can still become pregnant.

A low-dose oral contraceptive (for example the brands with only 20 mcg of estrogen) offers many health benefits apart from effective contraception. The pill makes periods regular which is a big plus in this stage of a woman's life. Hormonal contraceptives also insure a smoother transition into menopause because the woman herself determines when she has her last period simply by stopping the pill. If hormonal contraception is not an option, you can choose from the variety of methods presented in this book.

Family spacing

If you and your partner want to use contraception to delay the arrival of a child, the effectiveness of a method is not the main quality you are looking for. A natural method combined with the use of a barrier method could be a good choice for you. It requires knowledge and practice, qualities that will prepare you for the arrival of a new family member! Hormonal methods are more effective methods and the return to fertility is usually quite fast when you stop using them (**Chapter 3**). Another excellent alternative is the IUD (Chapter 7), provided there is no risk of STIs.

In sickness and in health

When you are sick and take certain medications you have to inform your health care provider and/or pharmacist about your contraceptive method. This especially applies to hormonal methods, which may interfere with the drugs you are taking for treatment of your health problem. The contraceptive may make the medication less effective or the medication you are taking may make the contraceptive ineffective.

Major surgery

If you have to undergo surgery, which will make you bedridden for a few days, and you are currently taking the pill you should stop taking it four weeks prior to the day of surgery. Don't forget to use another method during this time! If you had an accident and you undergo emergency surgery you should also stop taking the pill for a while.

This chapter is all about choices. We can only give you an idea. You have to discuss this in detail with your partner and health care provider to make sure you make the right choice!

ADDRESSES:
WHERE TO TURN TO

You need information, support? Here are phone numbers and websites that can help you.

Planned Parenthood Federation of Canada
Visit their website for additional information on how to be safely sexual. The site also lists addresses and phone numbers in every province. **www.ppfc.ca**

If you do not find the place where you live on the list, call the number near you and ask for the Planned Parenthood branch or clinic closest to you.

Alberta
Banff .... (403) 762-4511
Toll-Free 1-800-813-4138
Calgary (provincial) .... (403) 283-8591
Calgary (local) .... (403) 283-5580
Edmonton .... (780) 423-3737
Medicine Hat .... (403) 526-6111
STI/AIDS Info Line 1-800-772-2437

British Columbia
Vancouver .... (604) 731-4252
Facts of Life Line 1-800-739-7367
STI Info Line 1-800-661-4337
STI Info Line Vancouver .... (604) 872-6652

Manitoba
Website .... **www.serc.mb.ca**
Brandon .... (204) 727-0417
Winnipeg .... (204) 982-7800
STI Info Line .... (204) 945-2437
Facts of Life Line Winnipeg .... (204) 947-9222
Facts of Life Line 1-800-432-1957

New Brunswick
Florenceville .... (506) 392-5284
Fredericton .... (506) 454-6333

Newfoundland and Labrador
Website .... **www.wordplay.com**
St. John's .... (709) 579-1009
Info Line 1-877-666-9847

Nova Scotia
Amherst .... (902) 667-7500
Bridgewater .... (902) 543-1315
Halifax .... (902) 455-9656
New Glasgow .... (902) 755-4647
Sydney .... (902) 539-5158

Ontario

Websites . . . . **www.ppt.on.ca**
. . . . **http://planparenthoodottawa.on.ca**
Barrie . . . .(705) 725-9244
Blind River . . . . (705) 356-0113
356-2203
Hamilton . . . . (905) 528-3009
North Bay . . . . (705) 474-7762
Ottawa . . . . (613) 226-3234
Toronto . . . . (416) 961-0113
Waterloo . . . . (519) 743-6461
Facts of Life Line 1-800-463-6739

Quebec

Montreal
(For referral service in English language)
. . . .(514) 935-1004
(For referral service in French language)
Fédération du Québec pour le planning des naissances
(This is not a member of Planned Parenthood)
. . . . (514) 866-3721
. . . . (514) 522-6511

Saskatchewan

Regina . . . . (306) 522-0902
Saskatoon . . . . (306) 244-7989
Facts of Life Line 1-800-588-3228
Farm Stress Line 1-800-667-4442

SERENA Canada

For questions regarding natural methods call the National Secretariat in Ottawa. They can give you the phone numbers and addresses across Canada.
. . . . (613) 728-6536
. . . . 1-888-373-7362
Visit the website: **www.mlink.net/~serena**

The Kids Help Phone Line

A service with counsellors for kids from anywhere in Canada. You can call 24 hours a day, 7 days a week.
. . . . 1-800-668-6868
Visit the website: **http://kidshelp.sympatico.ca**

GLOSSARY

amenorrhoea: no bleeding during the time of the cycle when you normally would expect bleeding (menstruation).

anaemia: most common form is iron-deficiency anemia caused by the loss of too much blood. Anemia is lack of red blood cells.

cervical cancer: cancer of the cervix.

cervix: the entrance of the uterus, the passage between uterus and vagina.

EC: emergency contraception; methods described in Chapter 8.

ectopic pregnancy: an emergency situation, pregnancy outside the uterus, for example in the fallopian tubes.

endometrial cancer: cancer (abnormal cell growth) of the lining of the uterus.

endometriosis: inflammation of the endometrium. The tissue that makes the lining of the uterus can also grow elsewhere outside the uterus, which can lead to pain during menstruation and more blood loss than usual.

endometrium: lining of the uterus.

estrogen: female hormone, produced mainly in the ovaries. In its synthetic form (ethinyl estradiol) it is used as a component of oral contraceptive pills.

failure rate: term used in studies to describe the effectiveness of a contraceptive method. It is indicated as failure rate for *perfect use* (how effective is the method when it is used consistently and correctly?) and failure rate for *typical use* (how effective is the method when it is not used perfectly?).

HIV: human immunodeficiency virus, the virus that causes AIDS.

HPV: sexually transmitted human papillomaviruses, viruses associated with cancer of the cervix.

IUD: intrauterine device: a contraceptive described in Chapter 7.

menopause: the last menstrual period. Also: phase of a woman's life when estrogen production slows down and fertility comes to an end.

menstruation: cyclic bloody discharge from the uterus, also called "period."

OC: oral contraceptive pill, also called the pill.

ovarian cancer: cancer of the female egg-producing organs.

ovarian cysts: liquid filled sacs attached to the ovaries that can cause strong bleeding and pain.

Pap: stands for Papanicolau stain. A routine test to screen for cancerous cells in the cervix as a prevention of cervical cancer.

pelvic exam: examination of the inner and outer female reproductive organs described on page28.

PID: pelvic inflammatory disease. Inflammation of the inner reproductive organs of a female, which can lead to infertility.

POP: progestin-only pill, a hormonal contraceptive described in chapter 3.

progesterone: hormone mainly produced in the corpus luteum (the follicle from which the egg cell emerged at ovulation).

progestin: synthetic female hormone, used for hormonal contraception, either in combination with an estrogen or alone.

speculum: tool used for the gynaecological exam. It allows the physician to check the walls of the vagina and the cervix.

spotting: loss of small amounts of menstrual blood outside the normal menstruation.

STD: sexually transmitted disease, passed on through sexual contact, also referred to as STI (sexually transmitted infection).

STI: sexually transmitted infection, passed on through sexual contact, also referred to as STD (sexually transmitted disease).

thrombosis: blood clots that can impair blood circulation.

unscheduled bleeding: bleeding from the vagina other than the normal period/menstruation.

uterus: also called womb.

UTI: urinary tract infection.

vulva: female outer reproductive organ, entrance of the vagina.

INDEX

Text references are in plain type, photographs in **bold**,
and illustrations in *italic*.

The Canadian Contraception Guide is based on the Canadian Consensus Conference on Contraception and was developed under the direction of:

André B. Lalonde, MD, FRCSC
Executive Vice President, SOGC

Concept, Text, Project Management:

Elke Henneberg, Montreal, Quebec

Editor:

Carol-Ann Savick, Montreal, Quebec

Medical Editors:

Richard Boroditsky, MD, FRCSC *(Winnipeg, Manitoba)*
Terry O'Grady, MD, FRCSC *(St. John's, Newfoundland)*
Edith Guilbert, MD, MSc *(Quebec City, Quebec)*
André B. Lalonde, MD, FRCSC *(Ottawa, Ontario)*

Index:

Linda Cardella Cournoyer

Acknowledgements-Members of the Canadian Consensus Conference on Contraception 1998:

Richard Boroditsky, MD, FRCSC (Chair)
Edith Guilbert, MD, MSc (Chair)
Thomas E.R. Brown, PharmD
Dawn Bucharski, BScN
John Collins, MD, FRCSC
Victoria J. Davis, MD, FRCSC
Diane Francoeur, MD, CSPQ, FRCSC
Louise Hanvey, BN, MHA
Rosemary Killeen, BScPhm
Rena Kulczycki
André B. Lalonde, MD, FRCSC
Robert H. Lea, MD, FRCSC
Guylaine Lefebvre, MD, FRCSC
Carol McConnery, MD, CCFP
Robert L. Reid, MD, FRCSC
Timothy Rowe, MB BS, FRCSC
Louise-Andrée Saulnier, PhD (c)
Dorothy Shaw, MB, ChB, FRCSC